The SimplyRaw
Living Foods
DETOX MANUAL

The SimplyRaw
Living Foods
DETOX MANUAL

Natasha Kyssa

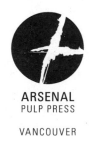

ARSENAL
PULP PRESS

VANCOUVER

THE SIMPLYRAW LIVING FOODS DETOX MANUAL
Copyright © 2009 by Natasha Kyssa

Second printing: 2009

ARSENAL PULP PRESS
Suite 200, 341 Water Street
Vancouver, BC
Canada V6B 1B8
arsenalpulp.com

The publisher gratefully acknowledges the support of the Government of Canada through the Book Publishing Industry Development Program and the Government of British Columbia through the Book Publishing Tax Credit Program for its publishing activities.

The author and publisher assert that the information contained in this book is true and complete to the best of their knowledge. All recommendations are made without guarantee on the part of the author and Arsenal Pulp Press. The author and publisher disclaim any liability in connection with the use of this information. For more information, contact the publisher.

Book design by Electra Design Group
Cover image from Photodisc
Photograph of Natasha Kyssa by Brendon Purdy
Editing by Susan Safyan

Printed and bound in Canada

Library and Archives Canada Cataloguing in Publication:

Kyssa, Natasha, 1961-
    The SimplyRaw living foods detox manual / Natasha Kyssa.

Includes bibliographical references and index.
ISBN 978-1-55152-250-0

    1. Detoxification (Health). 2. Nutrition. 3. Self-care, Health.
I. Title.

RA784.5.K98 2009   613.2   C2008-907776-8

In memory of my beloved brother Andre and dear father Yuri.

Contents

Note:

Foreword

Brian Clement, PhD, LNC, NMD, Hippocrates Health Institute

Natasha Kyssa's *SimplyRaw Living Foods Detox Manual* makes a major contribution to improving people's health. Her vast personal and professional experience affords her great insight and efficiency on matters of healing and preventing disease. The SimplyRaw approach also provides age-defying tools for those who would like to postpone their golden years. What is most important about her program is how easy it is to employ.

For decades, I have had the privilege to direct the Hippocrates Health Institute and other like-minded centers in Europe. In my experience, those who adopt a raw and living foods program gain renewed health and vitality. But, all too often, advocates of raw food complicate the subject with misconceptions and overzealous ambition. Natasha's approach is a breath of fresh air, based on her belief in adopting a lifestyle of integrity. Her leadership in the field of health and sustainability is respected globally and the major events she organizes to disseminate the message of self-motivation has swayed thousands to eat and live more responsibly. Natasha has more common sense than many who purport to be authorities on the subject of food and healing.

At this time in history, we can no longer afford to procrastinate and must take a stand to live our lives at the highest level achievable. Our food choices not only affect our own well-being, they also determine the future of our planetary environment. Building up our bodies with high-quality nutrients and cleansing them with pure methods improves our physical health as well as our greater emotional and spiritual well-being. The *SimplyRaw Living Foods Detox Manual* is easy to understand, easy to use, and a gateway to release all your past dietary offences. Henceforth, I will refer people to this important book and publicly thank this gifted teacher and author for her life's work, condensed here so that we can all enjoy the fruits of her labor.

Preface

I created The SimplyRaw Living Foods Detox Program after observing so many people "detoxifying" by taking various herbal and vitamin supplements, but not making fundamental changes to their diets. Detoxifying the body is an effective way to help bring it back into balance and positively impact your health. However, there is a lot of confusion about detoxification and healthy eating, and there are many products available on the market to support this confusion. Detoxification has become an enormous business, and there are hundreds of supplements, pills, kits, and books that make up a multimillion dollar industry. Sadly, consumers wanting a quick fix buy into this marketing hype, believing that a lifetime of toxins can be eliminated quickly with the right pills, while overlooking dietary and lifestyle changes. However, it is these long-term, constant changes that are essential for true health and healing to occur.

There are no quick fixes or magic bullets. Detoxifying the body does not occur overnight, nor is optimal health created instantly. Good health is an ongoing journey that requires perseverance, patience, and trust. Learning takes time. Stick with the guidelines in this manual, and you will achieve your goals!

It is important to understand that our bodies are constantly detoxifying. Cultivating healthy eating habits that assist this ongoing detoxification process throughout daily life is much more effective than a brief fast, occasional short-term diet, or use of any superficial products. Eating fresh chlorophyll- and enzyme-rich living foods will support this natural detoxification. In addition, you will be rebuilding your cells and health by eating these nutritious life-giving foods. By detoxifying and rebuilding the cells, we can achieve vibrant health.

The SimplyRaw Living Foods Detox Program focuses on health-enhancing practices to incorporate into your daily life. You will both cleanse and *nourish* your body with alkalizing, living foods, and you'll learn about many complementary cleansing therapies to help support your body's natural detoxification process.

It's simple, really. Eating live, natural, and whole foods promotes good health, and the more natural you make your diet, the better health you are going to enjoy. The body has an amazing ability to heal itself, and if cleansed and nourished with the right nutrients, it can repair itself. You cannot expect to cleanse and heal the body while eating animal products and other health-damaging foods, as these foods are highly acidic and mucus-forming. In fact, it is often the foods we eliminate from our diets that can influence our well-being more than the foods we add. To achieve optimal health, we must remove the toxins that hinder the healing process.

The SimplyRaw Living Foods Detox Program is based on my own lifestyle; lifelong dedication to and experimentation with fasting and cleansing the body; my studies with various teachers; years of leading detoxification groups through my practice; my work introducing friends, family, and clients to raw, living foods; and the many books I've read on detoxification, nutrition, and health. This manual has been inspired by the teachings of Dr Ann Wigmore, Paavo Airola, Dr Richard Anderson, Dr Norman Walker, and Dr Bernard Jensen, and draws from my years of experience with the raw lifestyle, fasting, and colon cleansing.

My transition to raw

Born in Montreal and raised by two very traditional European parents, I grew up on a very wholesome diet. Everything was prepared from scratch. Meals consisted of whole grains, large salads, vegetables, dark bread, and a lot of fruits. White bread, canned soup, and fast foods were simply not a part of our routine. We were not vegetarian but ate meat in small amounts a few times a week. So, as far back as I can remember, I always enjoyed and felt best when eating fresh and simple meals, with fruit, salads, sauerkraut, and olives as my particular favorites.

During my rebellious teenage years I moved away from home and fell into the trap of processed foods. As a result, I gained a lot of weight and started to feel lethargic, unhealthy, and depressed. Three years later (after gaining thirty-five pounds), I began working in my mother's vegetarian tea room and returned to eating natural foods. Adopting a macrobiotic diet quickly improved my health and stabilized my weight. It also eased the depression that I had struggled with off and on my whole life. This helped me to launch an international modeling career that would last over seven years, and propel me to a fast-paced, jet-setting lifestyle, globe trotting to exotic places around the world. Traveling between Canada, Japan, South East Asia, and Europe on a regular basis, I became consumed by the demand to maintain my slender model physique.

I soon developed a debilitating eating disorder that I secretly struggled with for over seven years, and was at one point hospitalized. Suffering from anorexia and bulimia, I restricted my diet to the point of emaciation, living on coffee, cigarettes, carrot juice, and a lot of algae—the latter two foods sustaining me. The effects were crippling, both physically and psychologically, as I was living a dual life of binging and purging. My life was out of control, my body out of balance, and I was lost in a downward cycle. I felt hopeless. This was truly a low point in my life.

During this period, I began searching for various lifestyles and alternative methods to help with my disordered eating habits as well as the emotional pain I had been numbing with food. I was painfully shy, and had difficulty communicating my feelings—issues I slowly began to address. I discovered meditation and began practicing regularly. I also discovered the writings of Harvey and Marilyn Diamond, Paavo Airola, Victoras Kulvinskas, and Dr Ann Wigmore, whose books validated my strong desire for raw foods. I quickly increased the amount of fresh raw and living foods into my diet and felt immediate health benefits.

It took a long time for me to reclaim my health, and I have since continued to refine this balance to improve my diet to what works for my body, progressing through many stages in my transition. Studying the Living Foods Lifestyle program at the Ann Wigmore Institute in Puerto Rico, I altered my lifestyle choices further to simplify my approach and to focus on easy-to-digest nutrition for optimal health. Spending time at the Hippocrates Health Institute in West Palm Beach furthered my nutritional awareness.

I also took up a variety of sports over the last ten years, a decision that's had a positive impact on my physical and emotional health. I am an avid runner and rock climber and enjoy leading an active life with my husband and son. Our favorite weekend activities are hiking in the local parkland, or snowshoeing in the beautiful and peaceful forest, away from the city. We also enjoy running along the Rideau Canal in Ottawa.

Transitioning to a healthier lifestyle has been an ongoing process for me, with many ups and downs. It has been an exciting journey and continues to evolve all the time. The living foods lifestyle has been life-changing for me, and after seventeen years, I feel more balanced and happier than ever before. I have found new ways of being—and continue to transform my life. I am grateful to have found this lifestyle and am pleased to be able to share my experiences and knowledge with you.

Throughout many years, I have experimented with various detoxification programs including water and juice fasts of forty days and more, yet I have found that the most effective program is one that supports the detox process in a gentle and consistent manner. I don't recommend harsh methods of cleansing because too-rapid detoxification can stress the body. It is also more challenging emotionally, and many people find it difficult to stick with such programs. As well, it can send the pendulum towards the opposite extreme, leading to sporadic and disordered eating.

While shorter cleanses can be helpful, they usually don't get to the root of chronic problems, which is why the SimplyRaw Living Foods Detox Program is one month long. Transformation occurs over time: twenty-eight days is long enough to break old habits and to create new, healthier ones. I recognize that it can be challenging to find the time to cleanse, so I developed this program to be simple, gradual, and realistic for you to incorporate into your daily lifestyle. It can be customized to suit your own needs, and there are many suggestions that can be used while travelling or socializing with others.

This program is about more than just cleansing the body; it's about cultivating the healthy habits that have the biggest impact on our well-being. It is also about awareness, personal growth, and reflection, empowering each one of us to make a difference to ourselves, our future, and our planet.

Whether you wish to have more energy, lose weight, clean your palate, or give your system a rest, you can make significant improvements in your well-being by following the guidelines in the SimplyRaw Detox Manual. You are about to embark on an exciting path of self-discovery and wellness.

Glowing health is within your reach!

—*Natasha Kyssa*

Acknowledgments

I wish to give thanks to my parents:

My mother, Ilse, for all the comforting times in the kitchen, as a child and adult, and for giving me the strength to pursue whatever my heart desires.

My father, Yuri, for exposing me to art, literature, languages, and culture, who was always there for me, believed in me, and loved me.

A special thanks to my husband, Mark, for his enduring love and encouragement. He continues to support me in this lifestyle and is a large part of my many projects. If not for him, this book would have remained only a dream.

To my son, Mischa, whom I cherish, who has tasted my many green concoctions, and who put up with me working frequent late nights. I hope to be a positive influence and role model for you.

A warm thanks to all my clients who have taught me, and who gave me feedback over the years, allowing me to fine-tune this book.

Thank you to the wonderful team at Arsenal Pulp Press for their invaluable efforts and superb professionalism: Brian Lam, Shyla Seller, Janice Beley, and especially my editor Susan Safyan, who has been most patient with me during this new writing process.

And to visionary Ann Wigmore, who pioneered the living foods lifestyle and who worked selflessly, helping many to improve their health by returning to nature.

Blessings to all of you who take this book into your hands and life; may your journey to better health be full of light.

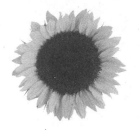

CHAPTER ONE

The Principles of Optimal Health

Introduction

THE SIMPLYRAW LIVING FOODS DETOX PROGRAM IS a gentle and effective program using fresh, uncooked plant foods to cleanse the body of accumulated wastes and toxins. The program isn't as restrictive as fasting and is easy to maintain during a regular working schedule. Unlike many other programs, you won't feel deprived or go hungry, and the abundance of vitamins, minerals, and enzymes will supply the body with the daily nutrients and energy that is necessary for optimum health. Instead of taking countless pills and supplements, the SimplyRaw detox invites you to participate in your own health by making healthy lifestyle changes.

The manual provides a shopping list, useful tips, health-enhancing practices to incorporate into your daily life, sample menus, reference materials, and delicious recipes to help transition to a living foods lifestyle. I recommend that you review the shopping list and purchase key ingredients at least one week before you start.

The SimplyRaw detox is a simple yet powerful program for improving your well-being on every level. You will have more energy and experience a lightness of body, mind, and spirit. Your immune system will be strengthened, digestion improved, and you will lose that extra weight and feel more positive in general. The lifestyle habits you learn during this program will stay with you for your lifetime.

Although you will achieve best results by following the program 100 percent, you may customize it to fit your own lifestyle and schedule. If you're not ready to go all the way, you may tailor it to meet your specific needs and still achieve positive results, making significant improvements to your health.

Our toxic world

"Chemicals … from well-known toxins to newer compounds with unknown effect are building up in our bodies and sometimes staying there for years."
—"The Pollution Within," by David Ewing Duncan, *National Geographic*, October 2006

We are living in a toxic and chemically polluted environment, and our health is threatened by the many chemicals and other pollutants in our air, food, and water.

Average people of all ages and races throughout the world are being inundated with thousands of chemicals that are invisible, odorless, and colorless, yet have a deadly effect on our bodies. Toxins include poisons, heavy metals, synthetic hormones and hormone-mimicking chemicals, pesticides, herbicides, cleaning solvents, and smog. These and many other substances are being absorbed into our bodies through contact with clothing, furniture, carpets, air, cosmetics, and the environment within which we live. Fortunately, our bodies are equipped with organs of elimination to clear away the accumulation of these toxins; however, when our organs are overworked, a buildup of toxicity occurs. Our health then suffers. We become fatigued, lack concentration, and become susceptible to sickness.

Many studies link environmental chemicals to the state of our health. Toxins disrupt normal metabolic functioning of the body, which, over time, can lead to conditions such as chronic fatigue, fibromyalgia, asthma, infertility, neurological disorders, and inflammatory disease. Cancer and cardiovascular disease, arthritis, allergies, obesity, and many skin problems are among the main toxicity-related diseases.

Toxins can damage our health, the health of our children, and the health of our planet.

How serious a problem is this? How widespread? How toxic are we? The report *Polluted Children, Toxic Nation* (*toxicnation.ca*) contains the results of "the first Canadian study to test for harmful chemicals in children's bodies, and the results show that Canadians, young and old, are polluted regardless of where they live, work, play, or go to school."

Toxins can be found in:

- processed foods (additives, dyes, preservatives)
- animal products (hormones, steroids, antibiotics in meat and dairy products, and mercury in fish)
- mold-contaminated foods (peanuts and cashews may be contaminated with aflatoxin)
- rancid vegetable oils
- tap water
- coffee and tea
- tobacco
- antibiotics and other pharmaceuticals
- pesticides, herbicides
- city air
- heavy metals in soil
- plastic products
- petroleum-based chemical cleaning products

- carpets
- plywood and particle board products containing formaldehyde
- dyes
- commercial shampoos, cosmetics, body care products, nail polish, hair dyes
- perfumes, colognes, and other scented products
- deodorants containing aluminum chlorohydrate, methylparaben, propylene glycol
- bedding (foam and cotton mattresses and pillows contain fire retardants and pesticides)
- candles with lead-core wicks
- soft vinyl floors
- photocopiers and correction fluid (trichloroethylene/TCE)

See page 60 for more information on making your home toxin-free.

How toxic are you?

The following may be symptoms of toxicity:

- exhaustion, fatigue
- muscle and joint pain
- compromised digestion
- intestinal bloating or gas
- chronic constipation, diarrhea
- recurring headaches
- arthritis
- cardiovascular disease

- excess weight
- sinus problems
- asthma
- psoriasis, adult acne, rashes
- abnormal body odor and breath
- coated tongue
- metallic taste in mouth
- food allergies

- brittle nails and hair
- depression
- mood swings and anxiety
- chronic fatigue syndrome, fibromyalgia
- poor memory or concentration
- frequent colds and flu
- insomnia or over-sleeping
- powerful food cravings
- environmental sensitivities, especially to odors

Tip: A strong body and immune system can resist toxic overload and disease.

Why detox?

In our toxic environment, detoxification is crucial, a matter of survival. We are assaulted with pollutants daily, from environmental pollutants to the toxins produced by our own bodies as byproducts of normal metabolism, and most of these toxins are stored in our bodies as acid, mucus, or fat. Toxins slow down the body's metabolism and lower immunity, leaving you feeling sluggish, heavy, tired—and ultimately causing illness and disease. Toxins can lodge in the organs, cells, and fat tissues, making it difficult to lose weight.

Our bodies are naturally equipped to eliminate harmful substances through the liver, kidneys, lungs, colon, skin, and lymphatic system. However, as toxins accumulate throughout the body, it can no longer keep up with elimination, leading to symptoms such as fatigue, headaches, aches and pains, coughs, congestion, and gastrointestinal problems. Long-term exposure can weaken our systems, increase our susceptibility to infection, and eventually lead to chronic illness.

To thrive in this increasingly polluted environment and to reverse illnesses, our bodies need extra support through detoxification. Many diseases are a form of toxicity in the body, and in order to reverse illness, we must first remove the toxicity. This can be achieved by eating a living foods diet.

Detoxifying is a vital part of any program designed to restore your body to optimum health and vitality, and can be one of the finest tools we have for our physical, mental, emotional, and spiritual health. The elimination of processed and acid-forming foods leads to reduced stress on the digestive system, allowing the body to focus its resources on healing.

As you rid your body of old toxic matter and provide it with an abundance of nutrients, the body goes into balance and does what it was designed to do—heal and stay healthy.

When the body is cleansed, it becomes more efficient at digestion, assimilation, and elimination. Detoxifying strengthens the immune system and gives your body greater energy. It also reduces inflammation and results in a slimmer body. Skin becomes softer and more youthful in appearance; your eyes sparkle and become brighter, you will shed excess weight, and you will feel much more vibrant, happy, and alive!

Detoxification also gives your body a much needed rest from poor dietary and lifestyle habits that have wreaked havoc on your health. When we eat an unnatural diet high in fats, meats, dairy, processed foods, and chemicals, detoxification becomes necessary, particularly to those who eat excessively. We need to cleanse more frequently and work harder to rebalance our bodies, depending on how far away from nature our diets and lifestyles have become.

The benefits of detoxing include:

- reduced toxic buildup
- increased energy and vitality
- stronger immune function
- improved digestion, absorption, and elimination
- slimmer figure
- blood purification
- reduced allergy symptoms
- clearer sinuses
- healthier, softer skin

- improved sleep patterns
- reduced cravings
- heightened mental clarity, focus, concentration, and memory
- better mental and emotional well-being
- a feeling of rejuvenation on all levels
- freedom from addictions to sugar, salt, refined carbohydrates, alcohol, junk foods, caffeine, nicotine

Why organic?

"Until we have a more complete understanding of pesticide toxicity, the benefit of the doubt should be awarded to protecting the environment, the worker, and the consumer—this precautionary approach is necessary because the data on risk to human health from exposure to pesticides are incomplete."
—*The British Medical Association Guide to Pesticides, Chemicals and Health. Report of the Board of Science and Education*, 1992

Organic produce has repeatedly been shown to be of higher nutritional value than conventionally grown produce. Toxic elements such as synthetic pesticides, fertilizers, herbicides, fungicides, antibiotics, sewage sludge, growth hormones (to produce meat, poultry, eggs, and dairy products) and confined-livestock operations are not permitted in organic production or certification. This means that there is a lower risk of pesticides affecting the soil, ground water, rivers, lakes, and atmosphere.

According to the Organic Council of Ontario, going organic has benefits for health, the environment, and livestock. Purchasing local organic foods brings an added benefit of sustainability as well as reducing transportation needs. Organic practices also aim to preserve biodiversity through the use of traditional seed varieties, crop rotation, and respect for the natural diversity of the local environment.

Organic foods are one of the most important choices we can make, and when we choose to purchase them, we are not only choosing higher-quality products, we are sending a powerful message by voting with our dollars. Organically grown foods:

- eliminate intake of chemicals and heavy metals linked to cancer and other diseases
- offer higher nutritional value than regular, conventionally grown foods
- protect future generations from widely used cancer-causing pesticides in food
- are not genetically modified (GM). It is currently not mandatory to label GM foods, and it is estimated that at least 60 percent of conventional food in grocery stores contain ingredients from genetically engineered crops.
- save energy
- minimize topsoil erosion
- protect water quality
- support smaller family farms dedicated to sustainability
- provide better working conditions for farmers and workers
- offer pure and natural taste (many top chefs use only organic produce)

If you must use commercial produce, always soak in a vegetable wash and/or peel well—but note that many nutrients are close to the peel.

Why eat raw and living foods?

Raw and living foods are high in enzymes that assist your body to digest food and absorb nutrients into the bloodstream. Enzymes play an important role in energy production and the repair of tissues, cells, and organs. They are the catalyst for life and are needed for every chemical reaction that takes place in the human body. Raw foods contain the enzymes required to convert molecules into the basic building blocks of metabolism: protein is converted into amino acids, complex carbohydrates and starches into simple sugars, fats into fatty acids.

In our modern world, our bodies are under stress from pollutants. To help combat the stress load and prevent disease, we need to nourish our bodies with easy-to-digest food. Raw and living foods are packed with the vitamins, minerals, enzymes, chlorophyll, oxygen, and antioxidants needed to fuel our cells.

When eating a diet high in raw fruits and vegetables, your body is able to focus its resources on cleansing and rebuilding the immune system. These nutrient-rich foods increase energy, assist healing, rebuild healthy tissue, and invigorate the entire body. You feel vital because all cell functions are operating at peak performance.

Dr Edward Howell writes, in *Enzyme Nutrition* (Avery 1995): "Enzymes are the catalyst for the hundreds of thousands of chemical reactions that occur throughout the body; they are essential for the digestion and absorption of foods as well as for the production of cellular energy. Enzymes are essential for most of the building and rebuilding that goes on constantly in our bodies."

Harmful effects of cooking

Cooking literally destroys the life of food. During the heating process, valuable nutritional substances are altered. Once cooked above 115 to 118 degrees F, enzymes are destroyed. Proteins are greatly altered, fats oxidized, vitamins diminished. Minerals undergo molecular changes at higher temperatures, making them more difficult for the body to digest and metabolize. Because cooked food passes through the digestive tract much more slowly than raw food, fermentation and putrefaction can occur, causing a buildup of gas and heartburn. Cooked food causes the body to work much harder for less nutrients.

Because there are few enzymes present in cooked foods, the body is forced to use its own limited reserves. Eventually, the body's own enzymes are depleted. Low enzyme activity has been found to contribute to chronic conditions such as diabetes, allergies, skin disorders, and cancer. It also results in weight gain, digestive disorders, lethargy, inflammation, and loss of both skin elasticity and muscle tone. Enzyme depletion and aging go hand-in-hand. Eating enzyme-less foods can also place a burden on your pancreas and other organs, which eventually exhausts these organs.

Studies conducted by the Hippocrates Health Institute drew direct links between a raw vegan diet, immune system recovery, and the healing of catastrophic illnesses and diseases.

Eat less, live longer

Aside from eating high-quality foods, eating less food is one of the best things we can do for our bodies to achieve optimal health. Instead of having a huge dinner, for example, you can break it up into smaller, more frequent meals and take the load off your body.

Studies have found that the majority of centenarians around the world typically ate much less than the average population. They avoided overtaxing their bodies and refrained from all kinds of overindulgences. All centenarians surveyed were moderate eaters throughout their lives.

Even the healthiest food, if eaten in excess, can make us unwell. The amount of food each individual needs depends on various factors such as gender, activity level, genetics, metabolism, growth rate, age, and climate. Try to tune in to your body and recognize your own true hunger needs. Genuine hunger is recognizable!

For optimal digestion, do not eat more than you can hold in two hands. Watch your portions, and eat only until you feel satisfied. If you aren't hungry, then don't eat. It's that simple. Be aware of realistic portion sizes and recognize that you may need to eat a bit more at first when transitioning away from a cooked diet as your body adjusts. Follow the three-quarters rule: stop eating when you are three-quarters full. The less food you eat all at once, the less hungry you feel because the food is more efficiently digested and utilized. Try to eat smaller meals and eat light to stay healthy!

Overeating

Overeating puts an enormous amount of stress on all the organs—especially the digestive system. In order to process a meal, the body must produce hydrochloric acid, pancreatic enzymes, bile, and other digestive substances. When we overeat, the digestive system cannot meet the demands placed upon it. This causes food to break down poorly, which leads to poor assimilation and absorption. Undigested excess waste also creates gases in the digestive tract that are absorbed into the blood, leading to a toxic body.

Studies show that overeating is one of the main causes of many degenerative diseases. In fact, overeating can poison the whole body. It diverts our energy towards processing food, instead of repairing, regenerating, and healing. Overburdening the body with food (even if it's "healthy" food) is not only a cause for obesity but other illnesses such as diabetes, high blood pressure, heart disease, and cancer. It also accelerates the aging process.

Most of us eat much more than we need. We are living in a very indulgent society where portions are huge, and we are conditioned from an early age to eat three meals plus snacks each day whether or not we are truly hungry. Our body wastes energy by trying to metabolize excessive amounts of food, leaving little energy to maintain health.

Most of us can easily reduce our food intake and be much healthier as a result. The best foods for us to eat are those that supply the maximum nutrition but require the least amount of work for our bodies to digest and assimilate. These are the high-water-content, chlorophyll-rich living foods.

If you must eat a large meal, make it lunch rather than dinner, as our bodies usually stop digesting soon after 8 p.m.

One of the first things people notice when eating a diet of nutrient-dense foods is that they don't have to eat as much to feel satisfied, and the cravings often go away. The cleaner your body, the more efficiently it will be able to function and thrive on less food, provided that it is high quality, nutrient-dense food.

Eating when stressed

Eating while stressed or rushed is one of the worst things we can do, as our digestion becomes compromised. Anything eaten during an aggravated state will either just sit in your stomach undigested or pass through the digestive tract undigested, causing diarrhea. Additionally, eating while stressed can trigger emotional eating, as we are not truly conscious of what we are doing during stressful times. This, too, can lead to further overeating.

Before and during eating, make sure you're relaxed. Avoid confrontations, serious discussions, or worries during meal times. Also avoid eating while driving, working, or watching television—especially the news. If you're stressed around meal times, allow yourself to slow down and relax before eating. Give yourself at least five minutes to unwind and take your mind off your worries. A few deep breaths in silence can greatly help reduce anxiety and tension. Light a candle, relax, and enjoy the act of eating away from the pressures of the world.

The importance of chewing

Digestion is the foundation of our health. The process of breaking down food into nutrients and absorbing these nutrients into the cells is critical to our health. If our food isn't completely digested, everything we do to try to attain optimal health will be less effective. Poor digestion is often at the root of health problems such as flatulence (intestinal gas), heartburn, burping, abdominal bloating, diarrhea, constipation, and nutritional deficiencies.

Digestion begins with chewing and mixing food with saliva in the mouth. We need to chew our food thoroughly, breaking it down into smaller particles and mixing it with our saliva. Human saliva contains enzymes. These enzymes (amylase) are produced by the salivary glands and break down starches into smaller molecules. The smaller the particles of food swallowed, the better broken down they will be in the stomach and the better nutrient absorption will be in the small intestine.

To get the most out of your food, you must be able to break down and effectively absorb the nutrients from the food. This means chewing food until it is completely liquefied. Why invest extra time and more money into preparing high-quality organic foods if you eat them hastily and forget to chew?

Maintaining a healthy weight

Often, people following a raw lifestyle do not lose weight, and some even gain pounds. This is usually due to overeating the wrong type of raw foods, such as nuts, seeds, and dehydrated foods, which are dense in calories and lacking in water. A nut-and-seed-based diet is between 70 to 90 percent fat. All fat is difficult to digest—more so than protein and carbohydrates. Cooked fats are even more difficult. Additionally, when excess calories are consumed beyond the body's needs, the body has to work harder. This contributes to excess free radicals (cellular damage) and aging.

Soaking nuts and seeds releases the enzyme inhibitors, and they become easier to digest, and less calorie-dense.

If you want to lose weight and be healthier in general, focus on high-water-content, quick-transit foods such as fresh fruits and vegetables with a moderate amount of fat. These foods provide the body with maximum nutrition and healing while demanding the least amount of time for digestion.

It is healthier to eat lightly steamed vegetables than to overeat nuts.

Weight-loss inhibitors:

- excess food intake
- excess fat intake
- lack of enzymes
- lack of high-water-content foods
- excess dehydrated foods
- lack of exercise
- late-night eating
- poor digestive, adrenal, or metabolic functions
- thyroid problems
- water retention
- sluggish liver
- mineral and vitamin deficiencies
- clogged colon, bowel difficulties
- yeast overgrowth
- food allergies
- parasites causing excessive appetite
- insulin imbalances

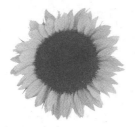

CHAPTER TWO

Getting Ready to Detox

"The doctor of the future will give no medicine, but will interest his [or her] patients in the care of the human frame, in his [or her] diet, and in the cause and prevention of disease."
—Thomas Edison

The SimplyRaw Living Foods Detox Program provides you with a week-by-week program outline, food lists, recipes, and recommendations for other complementary ways to enhance your detoxification process. A gradual approach is used in order to help you ease into the program. The essence of this program is to consume raw and living foods; however, a gentler option of eating lightly steamed vegetables at dinner is offered throughout the course. Although you will achieve best results by following the program 100 percent, you may customize it to fit your own lifestyle and schedule, and progress at your own pace.

The Progress Chart (page 73) should be filled out regularly to monitor detox symptoms, challenges, and positive changes. A food log or journal is also recommended to take inventory of your thoughts and feelings throughout your journey.

This four-week program is a basic outline and can be personalized to meet your specific needs. Each week a new set of goals will challenge you to bring your detox to a deeper level. If you can't go all the way, just do the best you can. Proceed at your own pace, although you will achieve more from the program by following the guidelines in the manual.

This program can help you improve your health regardless of how poor your diet has become. Whether you're eating an unhealthy diet, overcoming a health challenge, trying to lose weight, or just interested in feeling more energetic and youthful, the SimplyRaw Living Foods Detox Program is a sure way to help bring your health to the next level. Animal products, refined sugar, and processed starches are completely omitted, and because of this, health improves considerably. The program helps clean the palate and makes the transition to a healthier body and lifestyle easier. It is also a great way to prepare your body for a fast.

If this is your first detox, make sure to ease into the program slowly. If you jump into it too quickly, you will be more susceptible to stronger cravings and detoxification symptoms. If you are consuming alcohol, cigarettes, coffee, sugar, wheat, or any other harmful substances, start eliminating them at least a week before the program to reduce harsh detox symptoms. During the program, you must eliminate all of these substances or they will defeat the purpose of the detox, and you won't reap the health benefits. If you cannot meet this requirement, begin the program at a later time, when you can.

About the program

The program begins with one week of mostly raw foods to begin eliminating some of the more toxin-laden foods that are detrimental to our health, and to gradually prepare you for the 100 percent raw and living foods weeks. Week two of the program eliminates all cooked foods to incorporate strictly fresh fruits and vegetables. The Gentle Option is for those who wish to eat one type of steamed veggies with the evening raw meal. Keep in mind that your body will not detoxify as thoroughly when eating cooked foods. The third week moves into 100 percent living foods packed with powerful healing properties. The final week will challenge you with three days of consuming only blended foods that are easily digested and assimilated by your body. You will then gradually ease off the program with three days of living foods.

To optimize your cleanse, it is recommended you receive a series of three (or more) colonics during the program. For best results, schedule one colonic (see page 96) at the start of the program, one during the middle, and one at the end. During my cleanses, I always make sure to have at least two colonics every week to help eliminate mucus and toxins from my body. This can become expensive, so if it is not feasible, taking enemas (see page 98) will suffice.

It is essential to drink plenty of pure water throughout the program to help flush out the kidneys, detoxify the tissues, purify the blood, and rehydrate the cells. Tea, juice, smoothies, and soups do *not* count as water!

Keep track of your progress in a journal to explore your thoughts and feelings, and to help you be aware of the changes that you're experiencing. It is easy to forget where you have come from, and this is an excellent method of charting your progress over the course of the program.

Appendix 1 is rich with tasty and easy-to-prepare recipes to help you throughout this program. Be sure to experiment, vary your greens, and try out as many different recipes as you can!

Cleansing reactions

Cleansing reactions or "healing crises" (also known as Herxheimer reaction) occur when accumulated toxins break down and are released into the bloodstream. Toxins often leave the tissues faster than the body can eliminate them through its various systems, and this is when a cleansing reaction occurs. Detox symptoms are an indication that toxic substances are circulating in the bloodstream. The more toxins you are eliminating, the more severe the reactions are, as toxins are being released. This is a natural occurrence and essential for healing. It is important to understand that detoxification symptoms are the same as those of toxin accumulation. Toxins poison the body twice: going in as well as out!

You may feel ill; however, this will pass and you will feel much better once the toxins have been eliminated. It isn't always a comfortable process, and detoxification doesn't occur overnight, but if you remain on the program, cleansing reactions will become fewer and milder.

During the program (and especially during the first few days) you may experience some of the symptoms listed below. In fact, you may temporarily feel worse than you did before starting your cleanse. Try to see this as a good sign—and please be patient. Remember, we are carrying a lifetime of accumulated poisons in our bodies, and cleansing does not occur instantaneously.

As toxins are released, you may experience the following symptoms:

- headaches
- fevers and/or colds
- nausea
- coated tongue
- skin eruptions

- tiredness
- muscle aches
- lack of concentration
- weakness or dizziness
- mucus or other discharge

- short intervals of diarrhea
- constipation
- bloating
- frequent urination
- sugar cravings

- mood swings
- nervousness and irritability
- depression and negativity
- emotional upheaval

Symptoms shouldn't be suppressed with pain killers or antibiotics as this counteracts your body's natural cleansing process and compromises the immune system. If you regularly consume pain killers or digestive aids, stop taking them during the cleanse. These are the kinds of toxins that you want to remove from your system during a detox program, not put in. Detoxification allows healing, and this often takes time.

To help release these toxins, keep your system well-hydrated, drinking plenty of water throughout the day. To slow down severe cleansing reactions at any time during the program, you may eat a small bowl of lightly steamed mono (only one type of) vegetables.

Steamed vegetables will increase the workload required for digestion, assimilation, and elimination, and because they are cooked, the nutrient value is decreased.

Toxic emotions

Often, when toxins are being eliminated from your system, old and deeply suppressed emotions and unpleasant memories may surface. Most of us don't want to feel these negative emotions, so we may respond to these feelings by avoiding them, ignoring them, pretending they don't exist, or stuffing them back down with food. However, just like toxic food, negative emotions can make us ill.

When feelings are denied or suppressed, they become stored at the cellular level. This creates blockages and can often affect our thoughts, beliefs, and attitudes. Emotions such as anger, depression, or fear can also affect the nervous system's chemistry and weaken the immune system. Accumulated emotions in the body can build and manifest into the physical, leading to an acidic body, anxiety, heart disease, liver or lung trouble, and sometimes even cancer.

In order for the body to detoxify at its potential, we must also detoxify our emotional toxins. If you are holding onto anger, fear, resentment, or other negative or traumatic emotions, your detox process will fall short of its potential, no matter how raw you are. Releasing old, pent-up emotions is essential for the cleansing process—and for our wellness in general. It also gives us the opportunity for personal growth and can bring more joy into our life.

Resolving past issues can be challenging, especially when the problem is a long-standing one. The results, however, are worth the effort. Use this opportunity to write in your journal. As emotions arise, try to relax, observe, and identify the feelings. Allow yourself to *feel* these emotions. Be patient, acknowledge and forgive, and simply let it go.

Essential elements of the SimplyRaw program

The Living Foods Lifestyle (LFL) is a natural health program developed by Dr Ann Wigmore specifically for rebuilding and maintaining health. The LFL Program promotes total rejuvenation of the body and mind. It is a holistic approach to life. Dr Wigmore believed that there are no incurable diseases if one lives in harmony with nature. Her thirty-five years of research indicates that disease is a result of toxicity and deficiency caused by excessive cooked and processed foods, drugs, pollutants, and negative attitudes.

Living foods are provided by nature, organically grown, and consumed in their original, uncooked state. They are the most nutritious of all raw plant foods. Living foods include fresh fruits, vegetables, nuts, seeds, legumes, and grains, all prepared for optimal digestion by sprouting, blending, and fermenting. When eaten daily, these high-enzyme and oxygen-rich foods provide the body with life-giving, easy-to-digest nourishment. The chlorophyll content of Energy Soup, wheatgrass, salad greens, and sprouts helps restore and strengthen a weakened immune system. These nutrient-dense foods combat deficiencies and address problems of toxicity. When the body isn't using all its energy to digest food, it can focus its resources on other tasks, such as releasing stored toxins and healing.

Ann Wigmore (1909–1994)

Born in Lithuania, Ann Wigmore was a holistic health practitioner, nutritionist, teacher, author, whole foods advocate, and Living Foods Lifestyle founder. She was an early pioneer in the use of wheatgrass juice[1] and living foods for detoxifying and nourishing the body, mind, and spirit.

Dr Ann Wigmore dedicated her life to educating the world about the transforming qualities of the Living Foods Lifestyle. In her autobiography, *Why Suffer: How I Overcame Illness and Pain Naturally* (Avery, 1985), Ann tells of growing up in war-torn Lithuania. She was raised by her grandmother who exposed her to herbs and natural remedies as she observed her using them to help heal wounded World War I soldiers.

---

1. High in minerals, amino acids, enzymes, and Vitamins A, B-complex, C, E, and K, wheatgrass juice is helpful in building the immune system.

In her mid-teens, Ann joined the rest of her family in America where she quickly adopted the "new world's" eating habits and customs. She had a disastrous automobile accident that crushed her legs, resulting in gangrene. The doctors recommended amputation of both legs, but Ann refused, although her family sided with the doctors.

She soon reverted back to her grandmother's natural ways of healing, spending endless hours in her backyard in the sun, eating everything green she could find, mostly herbs, weeds, and grass, applying them also to her wounds. Slowly she regained her strength and eventually returned to her doctor, her wounds gone and legs healed. She recalls that the doctors "made no comment when X-ray films showed that the bones had knitted firmly."

Later, when diagnosed with colon cancer, she stated that following an American diet had caused the cancer. Again, Ann applied various natural healing modalities. Within a very short time, the cancer was reversed. She continued to research and study various whole foods and diet approaches, which she said not only cleared up her medical problems but changed her life. After many years of experimenting with food, she found a way to grow simple and easy-to-digest indoor greens, known as sprouts.

With a desire to share her knowledge, Dr Wigmore authored many books and lectured in various countries. She was an inspirational pioneer in the raw food movement who promoted the healing properties of wheatgrass juice. She invented the wheatgrass juicer by adding a sieve to a meat grinder, thus making it possible for people to grow and juice their own wheatgrass. Wheatgrass, she found, was easy and cheap to grow, and it contained one of the highest nutritional contents of the grasses.

She soon founded the Hippocrates Health Institute in Boston where she offered the Living Foods Lifestyle Program, which included wheatgrass, sprouts, Energy Soup, fermented foods, and her signature drink, Rejuvelac[2]. The Living Foods Lifestyle Program also involved exercise, deep breathing, and spiritual unfolding. Many of her philosophies are as old as Hippocrates (c. 460 BCE–370 BCE), who taught that, if given the correct nourishment, the body would heal itself.

Her work at the Hippocrates Health Institute produced testimonial after testimonial from guests who had cured themselves of various ailments including high blood pressure, diabetes, obesity, cancer, gastritis, stomach ulcers, pancreas and liver troubles, asthma, glaucoma, eczema, skin problems, constipation, hemorrhoids, diverticulitis, colitis, fatigue, arthritis, and anemia.

In February of 1994, Ann Wigmore died of smoke inhalation during a fire that

2. Rejuvelac is a homemade, fermented enzyme-rich drink made from organic cabbage or sprouted grain. It is a great aid for digestion and elimination, and contains the friendly bacteria required for a healthy colon. It is also an excellent antioxidant. See page 36 for more information.

destroyed the original home of the Hippocrates Health Institute in Boston. On that day, the world lost one of its great humanitarians and natural healers. Her work, teachings, and memory, however, live on. Today, there are several Institutes in the US that continue teaching the Living Food Lifestyle program, such as the Ann Wigmore Institute in Puerto Rico, the Hippocrates Health Institute in West Palm Beach, Florida, the Optimum Health Institutes of San Diego and Austin, and the Creative Health Institute in Michigan.

Energy Soup

Energy Soup is the most important food in the Living Foods Lifestyle. It is the ultimate high energy, easy-to-digest nourishment made from blended sprouts and greens. Energy Soup is a complete meal and contains every nutrient that your body needs in a balanced form. Because it is blended, the nutrients are rapidly absorbed, enabling your body to cleanse and rebuild in the quickest way without burdening the system. Energy Soup was developed by Dr Ann Wigmore and has helped with many health challenges that people suffer from every day. It is used to both nourish and detoxify the body. Since it is easy to digest, it is vital for those suffering from allergies and digestive problems. It is instrumental for correcting nutritional deficiencies, restoring health, promoting energy and weight loss, and is very easily assimilated by the body. Energy Soup is the first step to healing and is optimal for rebuilding health quickly.

It is best to prepare Energy Soup as close to the meal time as possible to keep it fresh. If using Rejuvelac (see page 36), Energy Soup can be eaten up to twenty-four hours after it is made because the high vitamin E content in Rejuvelac slows down oxidation. (If using filtered water, Energy Soup should be consumed within six hours.)

The following is a list of basic ingredients, used only as a guideline (see full recipe in Appendix 1, page 135). Use your own judgment and allow for creativity, but always include these basic ingredients. The recipe can be made for dinner, and leftovers stored in the fridge for the following day's breakfast or lunch.

- 1 tbsp seaweed (dulse)[3]
- 1 cup water or Rejuvelac
- small handful bean sprouts (mung, green peas, or lentils)
- large handful organic greens (spinach, kale, collard, chard, purslane, dandelion, watercress, parsley, etc.)
- large handful of sunflower greens (sprouts)

---

3. A sea vegetable, dulse is an excellent source of trace elements and iodine.

- small handful of buckwheat greens (sprouts)
- handful of alfalfa, fenugreek, or clover sprouts
- peeled apple, pear, papaya, or piece of watermelon
- avocado (use avocado only when nuts and seed dishes are not eaten at the same meal)

Pour one cup water or Rejuvelac (see page 36) into blender with the tablespoon of dulse. Do not overblend. Gradually add the rest of the ingredients, beginning with harder vegetables first. Leave sprouts and avocado for last. (Makes four servings).

Extras:
- leafy greens (for more chlorophyll to cleanse and rebuild blood and cells)
- cilantro, dill, basil, herbs

The most important elements, and the ones you should use in the largest quantity, are the sunflower sprouts. (Ann Wigmore called these "greens.") Instead of using avocado for the fat, you can use Flax Cream (see recipe in Appendix 1).

Sweeten your children's Energy Soup with a whole-food sugar, such as banana, apple, or fresh apple juice. Energy Soup topped with chopped or blended papaya makes it more palatable for kids. Diced avocado, green onions, and/or tomatoes give Energy Soup different textures and flavor. Experiment, and don't forget to chew your soup!

Nutritious ingredients in Energy Soup

Rejuvelac: Contains vitamins B, C, E, friendly bacteria, and enzymes for digestion. Rejuvelac prevents Energy Soup from oxidizing and enables you to keep your high-energy nourishment throughout the day.

Dulse: Any seaweed can be used, though dulse is preferred for the nutrition and taste. Dulse and kelp contain all the trace elements and minerals that we know of. Seaweeds provide some vitamins and are a great source of organic iodine. Using seaweeds ensures that you will be getting all of your trace elements and minerals in a balanced form.

Sprouts: Mung beans, lentils, and green peas (whole green peas and lentils, not split peas or split lentils). Mung beans contain protein, vitamin C, iron, potassium, and other valuable elements. Lentils provide protein, iron, and vitamin C. Green peas provide carbohydrates, vitamin A, iron, potassium, magnesium, and vitamin C. Sprouts are loaded with enzymes and oxygen, which make them a high-energy food. Sprouts also contain high amounts of fiber. In the sprouting process, the nutritional elements in sprouts are predigested, making them an easy-to-digest food.

Leafy greens: Healthy, organic greens are our connecting link to earth. All life comes from healthy Mother Earth. Only fresh, organically grown food has the capacity to rebuild diseased bodies. Leafy greens are high in essential minerals and chlorophyll. Any healthy organic greens can be used—including watercress, turnip greens, spinach, endive, escarole, lambsquarter, purslane, and dandelion.

Buckwheat greens or sprouts: These greens are an excellent source of chlorophyll, vitamins A and C, calcium, and lecithin. Buckwheat lecithin contains natural phosphorus and is a fat solvent. This means it is very effective as a way of removing fatty deposits from the tissues and cholesterol from the hardened arteries.

Sunflower greens: These sprouts will eventually grow into large sunflower plants. They contain an excellent balance of protein, chlorophyll, B-complex vitamins, vitamin E, calcium, iron, potassium, magnesium, and phosphorus. These greens have a very strong nutritional value and should be consumed daily.

Avocados: Avocados are an ideal food because they are a complete food. They are packed with nutrition and contain vitamins A, B_1, B_2, B_3, and generous portions of such minerals as iron, phosphorus, and magnesium. Avocados are about 12 percent oil and 8 percent carbohydrate—more like a nut than a fruit. The essential fatty acids in avocados are unrefined and beneficial to the body.

Apples: Apples mix well with vegetables, especially when used in a blended recipe. Apples contain protein, fat, carbohydrates, calcium, phosphorus, iron, sodium, potassium, vitamins A, B_1 and B_2, niacin, and C. They provide necessary natural sugars. (If papaya is used in place of apples in your Energy Soup, you will have about the same nutrients but will be adding valuable digestive enzymes.) Always peel non-organically grown apples and remove cores.

Rejuvelac

Rejuvelac is a fermented, enzyme-rich drink made from sprouted grains. It's a great aid for digestion and elimination, due to the fermentation process. Rejuvelac is one of the three most important items on the Living Foods Lifestyle Program, along with Energy Soup and wheatgrass juice. It is an excellent source of vitamins B, C, E, amino acids, simple sugars, and enzymes. Since it is a fermented food, Rejuvelac is also used for improving bowel flora.

Rejuvelac replaces the missing enzymes that cooked foods have destroyed. Because one of the biggest health problems is a deficiency of enzymes, Rejuvelac plays a vital role in restoring good health. Rejuvelac contains all the nutritional nourishment of wheat, is easily digested, and also works as an appetite suppressant. Although a beverage, Rejuvelac is actually so nutritious it could be classified as a food by itself.

HOW TO MAKE REJUVELAC

- 1 cup soft or hard wheat berries (or rye, kamut, or quinoa)
- 2 cups purified water
- 2 wide-mouthed Mason jars

Two reasons Rejuvelac works:

Reduces toxicity—A healthy colon is the most important means for eliminating toxins. If your colon is not functioning properly, you are toxic. The healthy bacteria in Rejuvelac and other fermented foods enable the colon to function properly by introducing healthy lactobacteria.

Rich in enzymes—The biggest deficiency most people now face is a deficiency of enzymes. Rejuvelac has a very high level of enzymes and replaces the missing enzymes in our bodies, enabling the healing process to take place.

Avoid using tap water because chlorine will interfere with the production of the bacteria. Like sprouts or any cultured food, it is possible for Rejuvelac to spoil. You can generally tell if Rejuvelac is good by the taste and smell. It is a cloudy liquid that has a tart lemon-like flavor, tinged with a doughy, yeasty flavor. Rejuvelac should keep in the fridge one week. Drink in place of water or juice between meals, or add to green smoothies or Energy Soup to reduce oxidization.

1. Place wheat berries (or grain) in clean Mason jar. Add twice as much water as berries and cover with gauze, held securely with an elastic band to soak overnight.

2. In the morning, rinse and drain wheat berries well. Sprout by placing the gauze-covered jar upside down at an angle, and rinsing twice a day. Sprout for two to three days or until the tail of the sprout is the same size as the grain.

3. When sprouts are ready, rinse well and drain one last time. Add water to the Mason jar (about two to three times the amount of sprouts).

4. Ferment at room temperature for two days. Cover the jar with cloth, but do not seal! Rejuvelac is ready to harvest when you see a thin, creamy foam on top of the water, which is rich in vitamins and minerals.

5. Pour off liquid Rejuvelac into another jar. Refrigerate. Refill original jar (still containing sprouted wheat) with water, reducing the amount of water, as the grains are milder. Let sit for one day and pour off the second batch. Refill again with even less water for the final batch of Rejuvelac. Compost wheat berries. Refrigerate.

Note that the strength of Rejuvelac also depends on the climate (the warmer the climate, the faster it ferments). If you prefer a stronger batch in the winter, let it ferment an extra day.

When preparing Rejuvelac (or Cabbage Rejuvelac, next page), be sure to keep the Mason jars sterile, otherwise bad bacteria can also grow in the jars during fermentation.

Cabbage Rejuvelac

When lactobacteria are to be taken, the recommended form is that of Cabbage Rejuvelac, which is obtained by fermenting fresh cabbage. Cabbage is teeming with lactobacteria. No starter is needed—Cabbage Rejuvelac is made with organic green (or purple) cabbage.

Good-quality Rejuvelac tastes similar to a cross between carbonated water and the whey obtained when making yogurt. Poor-quality Rejuvelac has a putrid odor and taste and should not be consumed. Always use good-quality water when making Rejuvelac (distilled, reverse osmosis, or filtered).

HOW TO MAKE CABBAGE REJUVELAC

- 3½ cups purified water
- 6 cups coarsely chopped, loosely packed fresh organic cabbage

Add water and cabbage to blender, and start blending at low speed for thirty seconds. Advance to high speed, and blend for another thirty seconds until well blended. Pour into a clean Mason jar, cover lightly with a cloth (do not seal!), and let stand at room temperature for three days.

Strain off the liquid Rejuvelac using a nut milk bag (used for making creamy nut and seed milks or for sprouting and available at many health food stores). Refrigerate liquid Rejuvelac, and compost the pulp. (All the nutrients are in the liquid.)

Cabbage Rejuvelac takes three days to mature. It will keep one week in the fridge.

I don't particularly care for using measuring cups, which has delayed me from writing an un-cook book, and find that a much easier way of preparing Cabbage Rejuvelac is to fill the blender to the top with cabbage and then just fill it up with water and blend!

Wheatgrass juice

The third essential element of the Living Foods Lifestyle is wheatgrass juice. Dr Ann Wigmore popularized wheatgrass for its healing properties. High in oxygen, minerals, amino acids, enzymes, and vitamins A, B-complex, C, E, and K, it is very helpful in building the immune system. Wheatgrass juice is the juice extracted from hard wheatberry seed sprouts. This strain of wheat has been used for thousands of years all around the world for its healing properties.

Wheatgrass juice is also rich in chlorophyll, the pigment which gives plants its green color. The molecular structure in chlorophyll is very similar to that of hemoglobin in humans, and some health experts believe that when wheatgrass is consumed, the production of hemoglobin is increased. Higher amounts of hemoglobin in the bloodstream lead to more oxygen-rich blood. It is easily absorbed by the body and uses little energy for digestion. Additionally, wheatgrass juice is a powerful blood cleanser and can help remove toxins from the bloodstream.

- The vitamin and mineral content of two ounces of fresh wheatgrass juice is equivalent to roughly four pounds of organic green vegetables.
- Wheatgrass juice improves the body's ability to heal wounds, release free oxygen, and may play a role in preventing tooth decay.
- It creates an unfavorable environment for unfriendly bacteria growth and can help drain the lymph system, carrying away many toxins from all body cells.
- Wheatgrass juice stimulates healthy tissue-cell growth.
- Wheatgrass contains up to 70 percent chlorophyll, which helps to purify the blood, and it helps keep hair from greying.
- It can neutralize toxins and carcinogen in the body, and helps purify the liver.
- It can improve blood sugar disorders and digestion.
- Wheatgrass can reduce high blood pressure and may play a role in the prevention and curing of cancer.
- It is a complete protein with about twenty amino acids.

Why wheatgrass juice?

You can purchase fresh wheatgrass "shots" at various juice bars. Some health food stores sell trays and/or bags of fresh wheatgrass as well as frozen wheatgrass in individual servings if you can't get it fresh.

You can also grow wheatgrass (or purchase bags of fresh wheatgrass) and make your own juice with a manual juicer. See *sprouting.com/wheatgrass.htm* or *chetday. com/wheatgrass.html* for detailed directions on how to grow your own wheatgrass. If you don't have a juicer, try chewing on wheatgrass. (Do not swallow the pulp.)

Super foods

The SimplyRaw Detox Program includes sprouted seeds, salad greens, blended and juiced foods, wheatgrass, sea vegetables, greens, fermented foods, and moderate amounts of nut and seed "cheeses." These foods provide optimum nutrition in an easy-to-digest form. They are essential to the program as they both nourish *and* detoxify the body.

Both blending and juicing have amazing health benefits. Personally, I enjoy both equally and find them very complementary. I tend to juice in the morning and early afternoon, and then blend later on in the day when I am hungrier.

Blending

Many feel that blending is superior to juicing. Ann Wigmore popularized blending and ate approximately 80 percent of her diet blended. Unlike juices, blended drinks contain fiber, are balanced, and are complete foods rather than an extraction. Extraction (juicing) removes plant fibers. Carrots and beets—both often juiced— are very high on the glycemic scale. Without fiber to protect us from the sugar content, carrot or beet juice can raise our blood sugar levels. Fiber helps with elimination and binds with many toxins and cholesterol before being eliminated from the body.

Fruit has always been considered a perfect food; however, modern fruit contains a lot of sugar (fructose). Some health experts, including Dr Brian Clement, director of the Hippocrates Health Institute, have suggested that hybrid fruits[4] contain up to 30 percent more sugar than heritage varieties. Most people can tolerate only a small amount of fruit because of these high sugar levels. If you have candida, diabetes, or other blood sugar issues, or cancer, eliminate sugar and sugary foods from your diet.

Fiber facts:

US recommended intake for fiber is 30 grams per day

The average North American intake is 10–15 grams

The Ann Wigmore Institute recommends 50–70 grams

Chimpanzees consume 300 grams

The average fiber content in an 8-oz glass of juice is 3 grams

Juicing

Freshly pressed green juices are excellent sources of nutrients. They contain high amounts of vitamins, minerals, enzymes, trace elements, amino acids, and antioxidants. Because juicing removes the fiber, these nutrients are immediately absorbed and assimilated directly from the stomach into the bloodstream. Juicing is extremely valuable as it places no digestive strain on the body. It also allows you to consume a greater and wider variety of vegetables than you can most likely eat.

When juicing, be sure to focus on high-chlorophyll-content vegetables (cucumber, celery, sprouts, kale) rather than the higher glycemic vegetables such as carrots and beets.

GROW YOUR OWN GREENS

Sunflower greens can be grown without soil (in baskets or trays). However, for highest nutrient value, it is best to grow them in soil, and in natural sunlight.

Equipment needed:
• organic unhulled sunflower seeds
• Mason jar
• tray or pie plate
• organic soil

---

4. Hybrid or seedless fruits may be genetically modified.

Instructions:
- In glass Mason jar, soak one part seeds in two to three times filtered water for eight to twelve hours.
- Drain and rinse.
- Let seeds sprout for one to two days, rinsing and draining twice a day. (The goal is to have a small root before planting.)
- Spread organic soil in planting tray, about one inch thick.
- Cover the soil with seeds, making sure they are not overlapping.
- Water until moist (but do not overwater!).
- Stack with another tray, pressing down to ensure that the seeds are in contact with the soil. You may wish to add extra weight with a stack of magazines or plates. Keep covered for three days, making sure to keep the light out.
- Uncover, water gently, and place in sunlight.
- Water (or mist) as needed, usually twice a day.
- Once the greens reach about seven to eight inches tall, they are ready to be harvested.
- Using scissors or a sharp knife, cut as close to the roots as possible.

Vegetable-source protein

It is easy to meet your protein requirements on a vegan diet despite the adverse hype from the meat and dairy industries. All plant foods contain protein. Studies show that vegetarians get plenty of protein, provided that a varied diet with sufficient calories is followed. In fact, you'd need to be in a state of starvation to be protein deficient.

Proteins are made up of a chain of amino acids, which are the building blocks of the human body. They help build, repair, and maintain all cells and tissues. During digestion, protein is broken down into amino acids, which are then absorbed and used to make new proteins. The body does not use whole proteins—it must break them down into amino acids.

Protein is found in abundance in plant foods, which are the best source, offering easy-to-assimilate amino acids. Plant proteins break down for assimilation quicker than animal proteins because they are generally already found in the form of amino acids. Unlike animal protein, plant-based protein sources also contain healthy fiber, vitamins, minerals, antioxidants, and phytochemicals. Cooking denatures the molecular structure of protein, causing amino acids to become coagulated and reducing the amount of usable protein. In his book *How to Get Well* (Health Plus, 1980), Paavo Airola, PhD, ND, notes that you only need one-half the amount of protein in your diet if you eat protein foods raw instead of cooked.

Animals (such as cows) rely on plants for protein. Instead of getting this protein directly from plants, meat eaters kill the animal (who has ingested it from plant sources) and get their protein second-hand. The body must work hard to break down this animal protein into amino acids, causing it stress. Meat protein is in a form that the body cannot assimilate easily, or use effectively. As well, animal products are high in artery-clogging cholesterol, saturated fat, and toxic residues. T. Colin Campbell, PhD, author of *The China Study: The Most Comprehensive Study of Nutrition Ever Conducted and the Startling Implications for Diet, Weight Loss and Long-term Health* (BenBella Books, 2005) states: "Published data show that animal protein promotes the growth of tumors." Excess protein consumption can also result in the accumulation of uric acid, kidney damage, dehydration, overacidity in the body, inflammation, autotoxemia, and intestinal putrefaction, and may be linked to many illnesses including heart disease, osteoporosis, diabetes, arthritis, and cancer. A high-protein diet may also cause premature aging and lower life expectancy.

It was once thought that various plant foods had to be eaten together in order to get their full protein value; however, research has shown that this is not the case. A varied diet of high-quality plant foods provides all the protein that you need.

The popular idea that we need extra protein if we are working hard is myth. In the bestseller *Diet for a New America* (HJ Kramer, 2nd ed., 1998), author John Robbins points out that protein consumption doesn't need to be higher during hard work and exercise than during rest. Robbins writes, "True, we need protein to replace enzymes, rebuild blood cells, grow hair, produce antibodies, and to fulfill certain other specific tasks … [But] study after study has found that protein combustion is no higher during exercise than under resting conditions." He also quotes the National Academy of Science as saying "there is little evidence that muscular activity increases the need for protein."

Athletes (including body builders) do not need to increase the percent of calories from protein. Lean muscle tissue can be built when following a low-fat, raw food diet—the healthiest of all diets.

How much is enough?

Many nutritionists now feel that twenty grams of protein daily is more than enough, and warn about the potential health dangers of consistently consuming more than this amount. Research now shows that the high protein requirements previously thought necessary are outdated and incorrect, and that the actual daily need for protein is far below (twenty-five to thirty-five grams) that which has long been considered necessary. And remember, raw proteins are utilized twice as efficiently as cooked. A good way to determine which foods provide sufficient protein is to consider the percentage of our total calorie intake that should be made up of protein and then determine which foods meet these recommendations. T. Colin Campbell, author of *The China Study*, states: "According to the recommended daily allowance

(RDA) for protein consumption, humans should be getting about 10 percent of our energey from protein. This is considerably more than the actual amount required. But because requirements may vary from individual to individual, 10 percent dietary protein is recommended."

When eating a variety of living plant foods, you get more than adequate protein. The percentage of calories made up by protein in most fruits and vegetables is equal to or surpasses that of human breast milk, which is designed to meet protein needs at the time of our fastest growth. On average, 5 percent of calories in fruit are from protein. Vegetables have from 20 to 50 percent of their calories from protein. Sprouted seeds, beans, and grains have from 10 to 25 percent of their calories in the form of protein.

Percentages of protein in vegan sources:

• spinach	49 %		• cantaloupe	9 %
• broccoli	45 %		• strawberry	8 %
• cauliflower	40 %		• orange	8 %
• lettuce	34 %		• watermelon	8 %
• peas	30 %		• peach	6 %
• green beans	26 %		• sweet potatoes	6 %
• cucumbers	24 %		• pear	5 %
• celery	21 %		• banana	5 %
• potatoes	11 %		• pineapple	3 %
• honeydew	10 %		• apple	1 %

Excellent sources of vegan protein:

- • leafy greens
- • broccoli, cauliflower
- • sprouts
- • hemp seeds
- • sunflower seeds
- • flax seeds

- • chia seeds
- • sprouted mung beans, peas, lentils
- • algae, spirulina, chlorella
- • bee pollen
- • wheatgrass

Seaweeds, algae, bee pollen, and leafy greens are very rich sources of good quality protein. A bowl of uncooked greens or sprouts may only contain a few grams of protein, but you can digest and assimilate it all because it still has all of the vitamins, minerals, and enzymes intact. Thus, this protein is far more beneficial to your body than animal protein. Nuts and seeds contain protein but are also high in fat.

Super sprouts

Sprouts are one of the most complete and nutritionally dense foods available.

They contain all the essential amino acids and other necessary nutrients, along with the enzymes to help assimilate them. They are a live food because they are a living plant. Sprouts are a predigested food that is very easily assimilated into the body. Fresh and available year round in the convenience of your own kitchen, these quick-energy foods are full of the concentrated nutrients that help our bodies detoxify and rebuild the immune system.

Unsoaked nuts and seeds are indigestible and contain mucus-forming enzyme inhibitors that need to be released by soaking. They are also very acidic to the body. Sprouts help to reduce the acid-alkaline imbalance that might occur when cooked grains, legumes, and other proteins are consumed.

During germination, seeds become alive and undergo many changes, making these foods far more digestible: enzymes become active; proteins convert into amino acids; carbohydrates convert into simple sugars; fats convert into fatty acids.

Benefits of sprouting:

- releases mucus-forming enzyme inhibitors
- activates enzymes
- increases vitamin content
- provides high quality, predigested nourishment (vitamins, minerals, amino acids, oxygen, phytochemicals, chlorophyll, enzymes)
- renders seeds more alkaline-forming

Sprouts are:

- fresh and available year round
- fun and easy to grow
- tasty and versatile
- economical and convenient

Seeds may be sprouted by many methods. However, using a wide-mouth Mason jar and screen of some sort is the most straightforward method. Quart-size Mason jars are available at most hardware stores. This size is preferred because the mouth is the standard size of sprouting lids sold at health food stores. A cheesecloth or stainless steel screen can be used instead of the lid, but it can be messy and wasteful as the cheesecloth tends to fray and the metal screen can become rusty over time.

SPROUTING 101

Materials needed:

- seeds (organic, whole)
- purified water
- Mason jar
- sprouting lid (or mesh with rubber band)
- dish rack (for placing jar at 45-degree angle)

Basic instructions for sprouting legumes:

1. Rinse the legumes (lentils, pea, chickpeas, etc.).

2. Place in Mason jar and cover with at least twice the amount of purified water.

3. Cover the jar with a light towel and soak for eight hours.

4. Pour off soak water and rinse well with cool water. Place drained jar upside down at a 45-degree angle on a dish rack to further drain.

5. Rinse and drain two to three times daily. Continue until the tail of the sprout is the same length as the legume.

6. Sprouts will stay fresh for a week when refrigerated.

Sprouting tips:

- Sprouts need to breathe—do not over pack!
- Sprouts need water.
- Soak at night and rinse in the morning (do not oversoak).
- Large seeds tend to get soft and become moldy if left too long at room temperature.
- Sprouts are best eaten raw because cooking destroys a large part of the nutritional content.
- Add sprouts to salads, pâtés, sushi rolls, collard wraps.
- Blend sprouts into smoothies.
- Garnish plates with sprouts.

If growing alfalfa, radish, clover, or broccoli sprouts, expose sprouts in the sun a few more days and continue rinsing until they are green and chlorophyll-rich. Chlorophyll = sun energy!

"Ode to Green Smoothies"

Reprinted with the permission of Victoria Boutenko, *rawfamily.com*
(See Appendix I, Section 2 "Green Smoothies," for more recipes).

As the Russian proverb says: New is something old that has been long forgotten. This summer I re-discovered Green Smoothies. What do I mean by a Green Smoothie? Here is one of my favorite recipes: 4 ripe pears, 1 bunch of parsley and 1 big cup of water. Blend well. This smoothie looks very green, but it tastes like fruit. I like Green Smoothies so much that I bought an extra blender and placed it in my office, so that I could make Green Smoothies throughout the day. More than half of all the food I've had in [the] last several months have been Green Smoothies. I have so much more energy and clarity that I have removed green juices from my diet. (Juicing has been something that I've been doing regularly for years.) Green Smoothies have numerous benefits for human health.

Green Smoothies are very nutritious. I believe that the following ratio in them is optimal for human consumption: about 60 percent ripe organic fruit mixed with about 40 percent organic green vegetables.

Green Smoothies are easy to digest. When blended well, all the valuable nutrients in these fruits and veggies become homogenized, or divided into such small particles that it becomes easy for the body to assimilate these nutrients. The Green Smoothies literally start to get absorbed in your mouth. Green Smoothies, as opposed to juices, are a complete food because they still have fiber.

Green Smoothies belong to the most palatable dishes for all humans of all ages. With a ratio of fruits to veggies of 60:40, the fruit taste dominates the flavor, yet at the same time the green vegetables balance out the sweetness of the fruit, adding nice zest to it. Green Smoothies are simply the best-tasting dishes for the majority of adults and children. I always make extra smoothie and offer it to my friends and customers. Some of them eat a standard American diet. They all finish their big cup of Green Smoothies with compliments and are quite surprised that something so green could taste so nice and sweet.

By consuming two or three cups of Green Smoothies daily you will consume enough greens for the day to nourish your body, and they will be well assimilated. Many people do not consume enough greens, even those who stay on a raw food diet. The molecule of chlorophyll has only one atom that makes it different from a molecule of human blood. According to [the] teachings of Dr Ann Wigmore, to consume chlorophyll is like receiving a healthy blood transfusion.

Green Smoothies are easy to make, and quick to clean up after. Many people told me that they do not consume green juices on a regular basis because it is time consuming to prepare them and to clean the equipment after juicing, or to drive to the juice bar.

Green Smoothies are perfect food for children of all ages, including babies of six or more months old when introducing new food to them after mother's milk. Of course you have to be careful and slowly increase the amount of Smoothies to avoid food allergies.

When you consume your greens in the form of Green Smoothies, you can greatly reduce the consumption of oils and salt in your diet.

Regular consumption of Green Smoothies forms a good habit of eating greens. Several people told me that after a couple of weeks of drinking Green Smoothies, they started to crave and enjoy eating more greens. Eating enough of green vegetable[s] is often a problem with many people, especially children.

Green Smoothies can easily be freshly made at any juice bar, restaurant or health food store for the great convenience of health-oriented customers.

I encourage the readers of this article to start playing with Green Smoothies, and to discover the many joys and benefits of this wonderful delicious and nutritious addition to the menu.

Here are more ideas for your green creations:

Some of my favorite greens to add to Green Smoothies: parsley, spinach, celery, kale and romaine. My favorite fruits for green Smoothies are: pears, peaches, nectarines, bananas, mangoes and apples. Strawberries and raspberries taste superb in Green Smoothies when combined with ripe bananas.

Delicious combinations

Mango-parsley
- 2 large mangos
- 1 bunch parsley
- water

Strawberry-banana-romaine
- 1 cup strawberries
- 2 bananas
- ½ bunch romaine
- water

Pear-kale-mint

- 4 ripe pears
- 4–5 leaves of kale
- ½ bunch of mint
- water

Banana-spinach

- 10 finger bananas
- 2 handfuls of spinach leaves
- water

Bosc pear-raspberry-kale

- 3 bosc pears
- 1 handful of raspberries
- 4–5 leaves of kale
- water

Fermented foods

Fermented or cultured vegetables are rich in enzymes and lactobacteria necessary for optimum health. They are predigested foods easily assimilated by the body with a minimum amount of digestive effort. Fermented foods promote a healthy immune system and assist with digestion. They also help digest other foods eaten together with them.

During the process of fermentation, starches, complex proteins, and fats are broken down into simple compounds, thus rendering these foods more digestible and the nutrients more bioavailable. A less expensive alternative to probiotics, cultured foods are alkaline and very cleansing to the body. They are ideal foods that should be consumed with every meal.

Fermented foods also introduce friendly bacteria into the colon. The colon can then synthesize vitamins, especially B vitamins, as well as produce beneficial lactic acid. These healthy micro-organisms are helpful with various bowel issues such as constipation, diarrhea, or colitis.

Sauerkraut

Unpasteurized sauerkraut is an excellent food to eat every day. Not only is it tasty, it is rich in beneficial enzymes and lactic acid. It is also a good source of fibre and essential nutrients, including iron, vitamin C, and vitamin K. During the eighteenth century, sailors ate sauerkraut on long voyages to prevent scurvy, a disease caused by vitamin C deficiency.

Most store-bought commercially prepared sauerkraut products have been pasteurized. They also contain salt (sodium chloride), which can be detrimental to health. Do not use salt when making sauerkraut; a better source of minerals is found in sea vegetables. (Table salt is 75 percent sodium chloride while sea vegetables are approximately 18 to 20 percent sodium chloride.)

Preparing sauerkraut at home is simple and can be done without having to buy any special equipment. It is also cost efficient.

HOW TO PREPARE SAUERKRAUT

- 2 large heads of cabbage (green, purple, or mixed)
- 1 tsp caraway seeds
- 2 tbsp dulse, wakame, or kombu (soaked and cut)

To prepare the cabbage, remove outer leaves and place aside. (These outer leaves will be used to cover the sauerkraut.) Shred cabbage by hand or in a food processor. Pack the cabbage tightly in a suitable container. Many people use a large crock, but a large Mason jar also works.

Pack layer after layer tightly into the crock or jar. Sprinkle caraway seeds and sea vegetables as you go along. With a potato masher or hands, pound the cabbage to help break it down and release the juices. Make sure the juice covers the cabbage completely as this prevents spoilage. This can be accomplished faster by using a Champion Juicer (with the blank blade) instead of shredding by hand.

If using a crock, fill to 80 percent, making sure the liquid brine covers the cabbage. Cover cabbage evenly with a few of the reserved outer cabbage leaves and add a plate with a weight on top. (A clean rock or a Mason jar full of water works well as a weight.) Drape a clean tea towel over the crock.

Place sauerkraut in a warm, dark place for five to seven days. After allotted time, open crock. Toss out the outer cabbage leaves. The top layer may be discolored and may need to be scraped off. If you like the taste, transfer sauerkraut into clean glass jars for storage and refrigerate. Sauerkraut should last one month in the fridge.

If using the glass jar method, pack in as much cabbage as possible. When it is full, press down and add more. Make sure that the cabbage is submerged in liquid. Close lid tightly.

For the jar method, just unscrew the jar, test fermentation, and place in fridge.

Makes approximately ten cups.

Variations are endless. You may also add combinations of carrots, beets, turnips, rutabaga, cauliflower, zucchini, radish, artichokes, onion, garlic, dill, thyme, basil, or juniper berries.

Nut and seed cheeses

Fermented nut and seed cheeses are the best method of eating nuts and seeds as they are predigested proteins. They are one step beyond sprouting for digestibility. Nut and seed cheeses are a valuable food, abundant in enzymes, lactic acid, B vitamins, and amino acids. They have a natural acidophilus, which helps with the friendly flora in the intestines. Fermented nuts and seeds offer more nutrition for less work by the digestive system.

SEED CHEESE (WITH REJUVELAC)

- 1 cup hulled sunflower or pumpkin seeds or almonds (soaked eight hours, sprouted eight hours)
- 1 cup Rejuvelac

In a blender, add Rejuvelac and seeds, blending into a smooth consistency. Pour the mixture into a clean Mason jar, and cover with nut milk bag or cheesecloth, securing it with a rubber band. Do not overfill as the seeds will expand as they ferment. Place jar in a warm area (on top of a fridge or near a warm stove) and leave undisturbed for six to twelve hours. Do not leave cheese for longer than twelve hours as it may become rancid.

With a large spoon, remove the seed cheese from the jar without mixing it with the whey (liquid) from the bottom of the jar. Or you may pour off the whey by inserting a spoon down one side of the jar to form a tunnel to pour the liquid out. The top layer of the cheese may be darker. This is fine. Most of the cheese will rise to the top of the jar and may have air bubbles due to fermentation. The liquid whey will separate to the bottom of the jar.

Remove cheese (solids) and store in an airtight container in the fridge. Seed cheese is delicious mixed with fresh herbs such as cilantro, dill, and basil. It will keep five days in the refrigerator. Makes about one cup.

SEED CHEESE (WITHOUT REJUVELAC)

- 1 cup hulled sunflower or pumpkin seeds (soaked eight hours, sprouted eight hours)
- 1 cup purified water
- ½ tsp vegan probiotic powder

Instead of Rejuvelac, you can use a vegan probiotic powder from the health food store. Preparation procedure is the same as with the Rejuvelac. Makes about one cup.

SEED YOGURT

- 1 cup hulled sunflower or pumpkin seeds (soaked eight hours, sprouted eight hours)
- 2 cups Rejuvelac (or 2 cups water and ½ tsp probiotic powder)

For seed yogurt, use twice as much Rejuvelac as seeds. Preparation procedure is the same as seed cheese, but instead of removing the cheese at the end, stir the mixture together with a spoon to finish making yogurt. Makes about two cups.

Healthy oils and fats

Most commercial oils have gone through extensive processing. They are not cold-pressed but heat extracted, refined from their original state, and devoid of nutrients and fiber. Additionally, most commercial oils have already gone rancid, which is extremely harmful to the body.

Extracted oils contain high levels of fat, which can be extremely difficult to digest and lead to heart disease. Excess fat in the blood can also result in an increased demand for insulin, draining the pancreas, and eventually leading to pancreatic fatigue as well as high levels of blood sugar. This makes us susceptible to hyper- and hypoglycemia, hyperinsulinism, diabetes, candida, and other lipid (fat) metabolic disorders.

A few tablespoons of oil can quickly turn a healthy salad into a high-fat meal, especially when combined with nuts, seeds, olives, and avocados. Two tablespoons of olive oil contains 240 calories from fat—100 percent fat. Instead of eating excessive extracted oils, try to eat the whole food source such as fresh olives, avocados, coconut meat, and soaked nuts and seeds. These complete foods contain important sources of fat in a form that is combined with other essential nutrients designed by nature to accompany fat. Bear in mind that these foods are also high in fat and need to be consumed in moderation. A good guideline to use is to consume no more than 10 percent of calories in fat.

Despite the concern about fat in our diet, the body *does* require healthy fats and oils to function. The average daily amount of oil should be no more than two tablespoons per day. When eating oils, make sure that they are not rancid and that they are high quality, cold-pressed, and organic. Always buy your oils from reputable companies in dark glass bottles so that they won't be exposed to light, which can quicken rancidity.

The living foods lifestyle

How much water we drink, sleep we get, and stress we experience can affect our health as much as what foods we eat, as can factors in our home environment. Traveling, socializing, and the eating habits of family members may also affect how successful we are at sticking to the detox program.

Water

Humans can survive a few weeks without food, but only a few days without water. Nothing destroys life quicker than lack of water! Water is required for every cell to function properly. It transports nutrients and hormones throughout the body's tissues and system, flushes out wastes, regulates body temperature, and supports chemical processes in the body. Water moisturizes the skin from the inside out and is essential in maintaining elasticity. It is the single most important element for cellular integrity.

The human body is comprised of approximately 75 percent water, the brain 80 percent water. Each day we lose approximately three quarts of water (twelve cups) through urine, sweat, and breathing. This water loss must be replaced every day. When your body is not adequately hydrated, it affects your overall health. One of the first symptoms is a headache. Often people will take an aspirin when they actually need to drink a couple of glasses of water instead. Other dehydration symptoms include stiffness, brain fog, low energy, back pain, chronic fatigue, and depression.

Many of us are chronically dehydrated without even realizing it. In fact, people often mistake thirst for hunger and then eat when their bodies actually need fluid. Remember to drink filtered, reverse osmosis, or distilled (not tap) water frequently throughout the day. Don't wait until you're thirsty to drink water—thirst indicates you have already become dehydrated!

Drinking water during the detox program is extremely important as it helps dilute and eliminate toxin accumulation. It also helps clear excessive fat from the bloodstream and can relieve constipation. You must make a consistent effort to drink adequate amounts of water. The more water you drink, the less room your body will have to be "hungry."

Staying properly hydrated will enhance digestion, nutrient absorption, skin hydration, detoxification, and virtually every aspect of your health.

Please note that coffee, soft drinks, and juice do *not* count as water.

Bottled water is not necessarily cleaner or safer than tap water. Plastics can also leach chemicals into the water that can be harmful to your health.

A few easy tips for drinking more water:

- Upon waking and before consuming anything else, drink at least two to three large glasses of water. This will rehydrate your body after sleeping as well as assist the cleansing process.
- Schedule your water intake by making a conscious effort to drink a glass of water every hour or so during the day. You could even use a timer to remind you.
- Keep a water log. Tracking your daily water intake (one tick marking each glass) in a notebook increases awareness and encourages you to stay on track.
- Get into the habit of carrying a large water bottle everywhere you go to drink from between meals. Glass containers (old pickle jars, Perrier bottles, or Mason jars), stainless steel canteens, and Sigg bottles are safer than using plastic products.
- Keep a large Mason jar next to you when you are at work and sip from it regularly for proper hydration. When it's empty, fill it up again!
- Add fresh (never bottled!) lemon juice to your water. This gives water a nice taste and makes it easier to drink more. Fresh lemon juice helps alkalize the body and is an excellent liver cleanser. Lemon juice also supplies vitamin C to the body.
- Try adding some fresh mint leaves to a large pitcher of water, and let sit overnight for a refreshing drink.
- Invest in a water purification system. You will save money in the long term.

To determine the amount of water required, calculate half your body weight (in pounds) and drink that number in ounces.

Below are some examples:
- Weight is 100 lbs—drink 50 oz water (four 12-oz glasses)
- Weight is 150 lbs—drink 75 oz water (six 12-oz glasses)
- Weight is 200 lbs—drink 100 oz water (eight 12-oz glasses)
- Weight is 250 lbs—drink 125 oz water (10.5 12-oz glasses)

Sleep

Getting a good night's sleep is as important as following a healthy diet and lifestyle. It not only recharges our energy levels but influences our overall health and general well-being. Studies show that sleep and rest play a critical role in immune function, metabolism, hormone cycles, memory, learning, and other vital functions.

Sleep is essential to vibrant health. It provides an opportunity for the body to repair and rejuvenate itself at a cellular level. Sleep allows the body to concentrate on repairing and building bone, muscle, and tissue without being interrupted by the many tasks performed while awake. Mental well-being is another important health benefit we get from proper rest and sleep. When we don't get adequate rest, we are less able to cope with and adjust to stress.

Research shows that depriving one's body of sleep decreases the quality of one's life as well as one's longevity. Chronic lack of sleep can weaken our immune system and make us more susceptible to illness and disease. It can disrupt our health in many ways, including hormonal and metabolism imbalances, accelerated aging, high blood pressure, obesity, increased onset and severity of type 2 diabetes, memory loss, and more.

During the detox, make sure to nourish your body with plenty of healing sleep, and don't underestimate the positive effect that sleep has in maintaining and restoring health. The average adult needs seven to eight hours of sleep, especially between the hours of 10 p.m. and 2 a.m. when the immune system most actively rejuvenates itself. A good night's sleep can lift your mood, improve your physical and mental state, and refresh your looks. If you experience fatigue during the day, take a nap, and let your body work its miracle.

Exercise

Diet is very important, but a good diet without exercise will not result in good health. Exercise is crucial for building and maintaining health. It strengthens the body, tones the digestive system, helps the bowels move, and plays an important role in preserving bone strength. It is also excellent for the circulatory system and helps release toxins through sweat.

Exercise can make you feel optimistic, strong, flexible, and in control of your own life. It is a great stress reliever and helps reduce the chances of developing many chronic diseases. Exercise also promotes the loss of excess pounds and helps further detoxification. It speeds up the metabolism so you burn fat rather than muscle.

Exercise doesn't have to be boring—it should be fun! Whether it is a daily walk, a cycle, swim, hike in nature, jog, rebounding, or yoga class, make exercise a healthy daily habit that you do (and enjoy) automatically. Aim for at least thirty minutes of exercise every day. The commitment of time and energy will pay off in a much better quality of life!

If you are overweight or have chronic health conditions, see your health care professional before starting a new exercise program.

Stress

We live in a very fast-paced world, and many of us are dealing with high stress levels every day. When stressed, the body's instinct is to defend itself by releasing hormones such as adrenaline (also known as epinephrine), which can increase breathing, heart rate, and blood pressure. As well, adrenaline causes a rapid release of glucose and fatty acids into the bloodstream. Senses become keener, stamina is increased, alertness is heightened, and sensitivity to pain is decreased. This temporary instinct is the body's way of dealing with short-term emergencies such as leaping out of the way of a speeding car.

Most of us, however, live under constant stress due to the ongoing pressures of our modern life. Whether the stress results from a tragic event such as bereavement or divorce, or just the daily hassles of rush hour traffic or too much email, chronic stress disrupts the body's internal balance (homeostasis) and can cause physical symptoms because the body does not have a chance to restore its normal equilibrium. Chronic stress is often ignored until obvious physical symptoms appear. It can be damaging to our health and often leads to an acidic body, fatigue, premature aging, anxiety attacks, impaired sleep, and suppressed immunity. Numerous studies have shown that stress is a major contributor to many diseases. In fact, being chronically anxious, irritated, angry, or negative can double one's chance of developing a major disease.

Stress is an unavoidable part of life, and it's not so much the stress itself that is the problem, but the way in which we react to its causes. Everyone handles stress differently and finds different outlets to relieve it. Some people deal with stress in an unhealthy way (reaching for a cigarette, coffee, or beer), while others cope in a more productive manner (going for a run, practicing yoga, stretching).

Since stress is unavoidable, it's important to learn to live with it in a healthier way.

Learning to manage stress is one of the most important steps you can take to protect your health. If you don't know how to manage it productively, it can cause health problems or make them worse. Of course, it is crucial to know just what stresses us out, and to work towards removing (or at least reducing) some of the actual causes.

Healthy methods of managing stress:

- Identify the source(s) of your stress. Knowing what is really bothering you is the first step in managing your stress.
- Make time for yourself. Often we try to meet everyone else's needs while neglecting our own.
- When you start to feel overwhelmed, take a moment and give yourself some space.
- Breathe. When stressed, your breathing becomes shallow. Taking deep, relaxed breaths helps slow your heart rate, lowers your blood pressure, and eases anxiety. Breathing deeply also helps you get plenty of oxygen.
- Stretch. Roll your head in gentle circles. Stretch toward the ceiling and bend side to side slowly. Roll your shoulders.
- Crank up the music and dance.

- Practice relaxation techniques such as yoga.
- Meditate. Meditation can take many forms. You may do it by following your breath or by repeating a mantra. There are many classes available for all levels as well as guided tapes to use at home.
- Share your feelings by talking to friends and family.
- Laugh. This is your body's natural stress release mechanism.
- Bounce! Rebounding is an excellent way of relieving stress (see page 94).
- Exercise is an ideal way to relieve pent-up tension. It helps you get in better shape, which makes you feel better.
- Do something that brings you joy!

Did you know that sugar decreases white blood cell count, leading to a weakened immune system? Sugar also creates acidity in the body and promotes an overgrowth of yeast and parasites in the intestinal tract. High-sugar foods include honey and all fruits (fresh and dried), so please use these foods sparingly.

Cravings can also be symptoms of detoxification and can occur as the actual food being craved is eliminated into the bloodstream. This is temporary. If you wish to slow down the symptoms, you may do so by eating heavier foods such as avocados, bananas, or soaked nuts.

Emotions also play a large part in food cravings as we frequently associate food with certain emotions. In fact, it is often the memory associated with the food rather than the actual food that we long for. For instance, we may want a pasta dinner with a glass of wine at the corner bistro when it is the socializing (with a loved one in a romantic setting!) that is desired. The association between comfort foods and our emotional state can be challenging to break, and if our emotional issues remain unaddressed, our food cravings will continue.

Pay attention to your patterns and habits. When cravings arise, ask yourself whether there is some underlying emotional issue that needs tending to. It is important to make a distinction between emotions and food in order to effectively address our true life issues. Use your journal and take time to reflect on what is really going on in your life, and what your body truly hungers after. It may mean that you need some nurturing. Look for the emotional link to your food, try to understand if anything triggered the craving (stress, financial worries, relationship problems), and look for positive ways to cope with these difficult situations. Practicing this will help you understand what food really means to you. It may be a social connection, joy, or even love that you really need. A helpful book to read is *Feeding the Hungry Heart* by Geneen Roth (Plume, 1993).

Remember, cravings are inevitable. If you have a setback and eat something off the program, simply start up again. Try not to be hard on yourself—learn from your mistakes, but don't dwell on them unnecessarily. Instead, focus on the positive changes that you're making and move forward again, restating your motivation and goals. Use this opportunity to see how you feel, and keep this in mind the next time you have cravings!

Cravings can be challenging during any detox program and may take time to dissipate. However, if they do continue, then you should work with a naturopath or other health practitioner to re-evaluate your diet and ensure no nutritional deficiency exists.

Feed the real void in your life, and most of your food cravings will melt away.

Food and family

It is important to consider how you will involve other family members on your detox journey. Introducing this new way of eating to your family can present challenges for most people. Explain what you will be doing—and why—before embarking on the program. The key is to not force anything on anyone else. All you can do is set an example and let them see the positive changes in your appearance, health, and attitude.

Keep it fun and nonthreatening. Offer your family plenty of delicious options and health information. Have fruits, dips, pâtés, cucumbers, carrots, or almond butter on celery sticks available on the table after school when children are hungry and more receptive to new tastes. If they reject these new foods at first, keep offering them. Often they need to see them several times before they look and taste familiar.

Make food visually appealing, and don't announce that the food is "raw," as this can put too much emphasis on your meal and turn others off. Best to wait until after they've tasted and *loved* your amazing raw creations!

Having your children help out in the kitchen (i.e., rolling raw truffles, growing sprouts, juicing, making "noodles" with the spiral slicer) is an excellent way to gently involve them in your healthy new lifestyle.

Socializing

The most important guideline when going out is to always plan ahead and make sure that you have healthy food on hand. Dried fruit, an apple, banana, avocado, olives, nuts, seeds, dehydrated crackers (purchased from the health food store) or dulse can easily be tucked away in your bag to snack on or to enhance salads. It is also important not to leave home on an empty stomach as this will increase the chance for temptation.

If you are tempted, remind yourself that the pleasure you get from eating something off the program is only temporary and lasts just a few minutes, while the pleasure of true health derived from the detox program lasts a lifetime.

At restaurants, explain to the server that you are a "raw food eater" and that you would like a large tossed salad with extras such as an avocado, diced vegetables, and a slice of lemon for the dressing (if you didn't bring your own). You'd be surprised just how accommodating restaurants are, especially when you're polite about your special requests. Whenever I dine out at our neighborhood Mexican restaurant, the owner brings me a veggie platter (instead of the chips) to dip into the raw vegan guacamole. (Be sure to inquire about the ingredients in dishes being offered. I have often gone out for dinner only to find out that the salad is cooked or contains animal products. At a Mexican restaurant in Los Angeles, I noticed that the guacamole had an odd smell. When I asked about the ingredients, I was told that the restaurant used sour cream to make the guacamole creamier! Luckily, my sense of smell was good, and I caught it before dipping in.)

Even when invited over to friends' homes, make sure to pack raw snacks to take along with you as backup. It is better to be safe than to give in to temptation and later regret it. Bringing a raw salad, pâté, or dessert to gatherings is another excellent way of ensuring that you won't go hungry. It is also a great way to introduce your friends to the lifestyle. Don't be surprised if they start asking you to bring that fabulous raw carrot cake to the next dinner.

Raw traveling

Whether traveling by car or by plane, make sure to always go prepared. Bringing a few raw items along with you can make all the difference and completely transform your travels. A few days prior to your trip, make sure to consume a lot of green smoothies, fresh juices, and water, and remember to rest up.

If you are traveling by car, you will have more freedom and space to store food and light kitchen items. A large cooler (or two—one in the trunk, one in the front) full of edibles, a grater, bowl, cutting board, sharp knife, peeler, utensils, portable blender, assortment of containers, and ziplock bags for storing food are handy to have on hand whenever you decide to picnic along the way. Traveling by car also allows you to load up on fresh local produce at farmer's markets, fruit stands, and natural food stores along the way.

Flying can be more challenging with all of the restrictions and limits. I used to travel with green smoothies and juices but now bring powdered Vitamineral™ Greens for adding to water and chlorella tablets instead. For carry-on, be sure to bring an empty shaker bottle; once past security, purchase a few quarts of bottled water to mix with your green powder. Personally, I prefer traveling light, hydrating my body with plenty of water, and eating mostly high-water-content foods such as fruit, sprouts, or greens, as I find that being inactive slows down my digestion.

Before packing your snacks, be sure to check with the airline to ensure you can bring your own food past security. Useful snacks to pack in your carry-on bag are apples or other fruits (please note that some airports have restrictions on certain fruits), dulse, nori sheets, sunflower greens, diced avocado, sauerkraut, dried fruit, goji berries, and dehydrated crackers. You could also bring a small marinated kale salad for the flight. Bee pollen, chlorella tablets, Vitamineral™ Green, and enzymes are also good to have with you to assist with digestion. Dehydrated, seasoned nuts or seeds come in handy to snack on and are very easy to transport.

Please note that most airlines offer a fruit plate and, while not organic, it is a high-water-content meal, which is much easier to digest. Make sure to call ahead to reserve your special meal.

Essential travel kit
Check local air travel restrictions before bringing any food or food accessories to the airport!

- chlorella tablets
- Vitamineral™ Green
- chia seeds
- bee pollen
- enzymes
- probiotics
- homemade salad dressing*
- cut-up veggies
- a few apples
- dried fruit (goji, figs, apricots, raisins, prunes, dates)

- nuts and seeds
- dehydrated crackers
- raw almond butter
- dulse, nori, wakame
- glass or plastic container with lid
- portable or hand-held blender*
- nut milk bag*
- lunch box cooler*
- lavender essential oil (used topically for relaxation, improved sleep quality, and headaches)

*(if traveling by car, bus or train)

If you're staying in a hotel, ask in advance for a room with a refrigerator. It might cost extra, but it will be well worth it. If not available, you might be able to use the ice box commonly used for chilling wine—fill it up with ice, and place your produce on top. You may alternately wish to fill the trash can with ice, as it is usually larger and holds more. During longer stays, I have often sprouted in hotel rooms with my nut milk bag hanging over a tray in the bathroom.

When staying with friends or family, make your dietary preferences known in advance so there won't be any awkward surprises. Offer to make green smoothies and other healthy, delicious meals for everyone.

Making your home toxin free

Cleaning and personal body care products are among the most toxic source of chemicals in your home. Most poisonings happen slowly, over a long period of time, by daily exposure to toxins in the air and toxic chemicals that come into contact with the skin. Many of the ingredients in personal care products can be ingested during use (such as some ingredients in mouthwash and toothpaste), or can be absorbed through the skin into the bloodstream (soaps, lotions, creams, cosmetics, shampoos, deodorants, etc.). These products can be easily replaced with safe, effective, and affordable alternatives available at most natural food stores.

Remove toxic substances from your life and replace them with nontoxic alternatives.

Recommendations for a nontoxic home:

- Use only nontoxic cleaning and personal care products. Read ingredients listed and avoid toxic substances such as fluoride and sodium laurate in toothpastes and shampoos.
- Avoid scented products including all perfume, aftershave, personal care products, air fresheners, potpourri, etc.
- Avoid all fabric softeners, dryer sheets, and scented detergents. These products are very toxic and harmful to the environment.
- Avoid plastics and aluminum as much as possible when preparing or storing food. (It's best to store food in glass jars.)
- Drink and bathe in filtered water. Fumes from chlorinated water may be absorbed by the lungs. Filters that easily attach to your shower nozzle can be purchased from water suppliers or natural food stores.
- Eat organic food (food grown without synthetic pesticides or fertilizers) as often as possible.
- Avoid processed foods, which contain preservatives, nitrates, and dyes.
- Never consume products containing NutraSweet (aspartame). Some health advocates are concerned that it can break down into formic acid and methanol (wood alcohol) in the body.

- Minimize your exposure to mold spores and dust mites by keeping the ducts in your home clean.
- Use an air purifier or ionizer air filter to remove chemicals and toxins in the air.
- Remove shoes before entering the house to prevent tracking in toxins.
- During the day, open your windows to get fresh air and to dilute some of the toxic air. Even in the most polluted cities, outdoor air has generally been found to be less toxic than indoor air.
- Purchase air-purifying plants such as English ivy, spider plants, areca palm, peace lily, or Boston fern.
- Avoid particle board, plywood, glues, inks, foam rubber, vinyl, carpet, synthetic rugs, varnishes, and solvents containing potentially harmful chemicals.
- Avoid all pesticides, fungicides, herbicides, and fertilizers. Pesticides are neurotoxins and affect the central nervous system.
- Reduce exposure to electric magnetic fields (EMFs) by minimizing cell phone use and by removing electrical devices and cords near your bed. For example, use battery-operated clocks and move radios and answering machines away from the head of your bed.

Skin care

Cosmetics and body care products are often overlooked as sources of toxins, but they contain a significant amount of chemicals. Thousands of harmful chemicals are used in everyday cosmetics and body care products, which, with long-term exposure, can be detrimental to our health.

The skin is the largest organ of elimination in the body and has the ability to absorb substances it comes in contact with. In fact, approximately 60 percent of what we put on our skin is absorbed into our bodies. When we apply body care products (makeup, shampoo, conditioner, creams, soap, perfumes, lotions, lipstick, etc.) directly to our bodies, we not only ingest them through our skin but also through our nose, scalp, and mouth.

The beauty product industry has become a multibillion dollar business, and women generally use up to a dozen body care products every day, which can contain over 100 synthetic chemicals. Repeated exposure can accumulate and lead to severe skin irritation, eye damage, neurological problems, kidney and liver damage, and, potentially, various forms of cancer.

Make sure to inform yourself about the beauty products that you use, know which ingredients are problematic, and refrain from using nail polish, perfumes, and especially hair dyes as these are all known to be highly carcinogenic. Get into the habit of reading the ingredients on your beauty products just as you would your food. Many companies (including those found at natural food stores) claim to be "natural" or use "organic" ingredients; however, they often use a few healthy ingredients mixed in with synthetic chemicals and petroleum-based colors, fragrances, and preservatives so they can call their product natural. If you don't know what the ingredients are, a good rule of thumb is, "If you can't pronounce it, you don't need it!"

Chemicals found in some cosmetics and personal care products:

- alcohol, isopropyl (SD−40): eye makeup, bath products, aftershave, nail products
- aluminum: most antiperspirants, some lip gloss and liners
- benzalkonium chloride: shampoos, personal cleanliness products, skin cleansers, skin care, and eye makeup preparations.
- formaldehyde: nail polish, shower gel, liquid hand wash, and bubble bath
- lead: somes lipsticks
- lauryl sulphate (SLS), sodium laureth sulphate (SLES): toothpaste, shampoo, bath foam, body and shower gels

- mercury: eye liner, mascara, soaps, skin lighteners, eye drops
- paraben preservatives or alkyl-p-hydroxybenzoates (methyl, propyl, butyl, and ethyl): conditioners, hair styling gels, foundations, concealers, mascara, skin creams, deodorants, sunscreen, hair dye
- petroleum: makeup, skin care products, conditioner, bath products
- propylene/butylenes glycol (PG): deodorants, lotions, conditioner, gel, creams, lipstick, hand wipes
- pthalates: hairsprays, hair straighteners, body lotions
- talc: hygiene products, cosmetics

Many soaps and cosmetics also contain animal fats and oils including tallow, which has been derived from cattle. So if you're concerned about ingesting animal products through your skin, do your research before your purchase.

If you won't eat it, don't put it on your skin!

Rather than using store-bought creams, I like to use cold-pressed organic virgin coconut oil as both my moisturizer and hair cream. It also works wonders as a sun lotion. Coconut oil is good for you internally and externally; I always have a jar of it in my kitchen and bathroom. It smells good and tastes great!

Detoxify your kitchen

Before starting your new way of eating, go through your cupboards and remove non-raw items. It is important to keep temptations out of sight and mind as much as possible. Remove all processed or other foods that are not part of the program. If you live with others, make room for a special detox shelf in the cupboard and fridge.

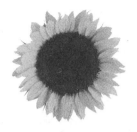

CHAPTER THREE

The 28-Day SimplyRaw Detox Program

GOING RAW IS A HUGE LEARNING CURVE FOR most people. The key is to plan ahead, making sure to have a steady supply of apples, avocados, sprouts, leafy greens, vegetables, and bananas available in your kitchen. Initially it might take more time to prepare raw dishes, but with time, you will learn shortcuts such as washing produce a few days before and having it ready for quick green smoothies, juices, and salads.

Personal goals and motivation

Often, people fail to commit to something because they are afraid that they cannot continue it *forever*. Throughout the program, remind yourself that you are committing to the program not forever but for twenty-eight days. This way, you won't be as overwhelmed or discouraged, because you're committing to changing your diet, not for a lifetime but for a short period of time. (Of course, you might be pleased with the end results and choose to continue with some of these new, healthier habits.)

Twenty-eight days is sufficient time to make a difference, and a short enough period of time to not overwhelm you, which is the number-one reason people quit or break their commitment. Breaking old habits and developing new ones take time. Remind yourself that this is for only four weeks of your life, and these weeks will have a long-term positive outcome on your health. You could commit to an exercise routine for one month, right? You can also change your eating habits. After all, it's only twenty-eight days. Although after completing this program, you'll look and feel so good that you'll want to continue with many of the guidelines in this book.

Find a friend to detox with for added support and encouragement.

Before you begin the program, write down three reasons why you want to cleanse. Make your reasons specific and achievable. Changing eating habits can be difficult, and many of us often don't have enough motivation to follow through. Ask yourself why you are doing this detox program. Are you looking to feel more energetic or is it those extra five pounds you're hoping to shed? Understanding your intentions will keep you motivated and strong. Be sure to use positive affirmations beginning with "I will" instead of negative ones with "I won't." Place your list of affirmations on the fridge or at your desk where you can see it each day. Use the power of visualization and see yourself as you want to look and feel.

Keeping a journal throughout the program is highly recommended as it helps clarify your goals. It is also an important self-exploration tool: journaling reminds you to be consistent and keeps you accountable. It helps keep you honest, clarifying your thoughts and feelings, thereby giving you valuable self-knowledge. It is important to express your thoughts, feelings, reflections, doubts, desires, fears, highs, lows, and insights that may arise during your journey. Pay attention to your emotional self; try to notice any changes in your mood or attitude. Negativity and pessimism often fade away and are replaced with an optimistic and more positive outlook.

You may also wish to keep a record of the food you eat, the amount and time of day, and how you feel before and after eating. By doing this, you will learn about your connection to food, your triggers and patterns for eating, and increase your awareness of the impact of food on your body.

Have fun. Embrace the process, the gradual changes, and yourself. You are making changes that will allow you greater health and enjoyment in the future.

Buddy system

Finding a friend to join you on your detox journey can help keep you motivated, committed, and strong. Having the moral support, encouragement, and friendship throughout the process will also make your experience a lot more enjoyable. Doing a detox program alone can be socially isolating at times, so it's great to have a buddy to check in, share laughs, and compare notes with, someone with whom you can spend time in the kitchen. This is definitely a bonding experience!

Getting started (one week before)

Give yourself at least one week to prepare for the program. The gentlest way to transition is to slowly remove the more processed foods a week or two before beginning the complete detox. Reduce coffee, meat, white flour, and sugar by half, and then a few days later, eliminate them altogether.

At the same time, begin introducing fresh, raw foods into your diet. Make wheatgrass or E₃Live[1] part of your morning ritual, and consume fruit and green smoothies daily. This can also be started the week before beginning the full program (or earlier), depending on your schedule and needs.

Tips in the kitchen

- Always plan ahead. Buy bananas and avocados in advance to ensure that you'll have ripe ones every day. Place on top of fridge or in paper bag to ripen.
- After grocery shopping, wash vegetables and put in sealed containers in fridge.
- Wash leafy greens in advance. This will cut down your prep time in the kitchen and motivate you to make green smoothies, juices, and salads. When ripe (soft to the touch) place avocados in the fridge to keep longer.
- Soak nuts and seeds before going to bed. In the morning, rinse, drain, and refrigerate, or use immediately.
- To save time in the morning, make a large batch of plain nut milk the night before. (This will keep three days in the fridge.) In the morning, add fruit and sweetener only to the amount you will consume that day.
- When making salad dressings, make extra to use throughout the week.
- Purchase pre-washed organic greens for quick salads or green smoothies.
- Prepare large fruit salads to have on hand for snacking.
- Make pesto and marinara sauce and freeze in small jars.
- Prepare large batches of sunflower pâté ahead of time. Use in various ways: for wraps, sushi rolls, stuffed peppers, or on salads.
- When hungry and on-the-go, eat a ripe banana or apple.
- Always pack a handful of soaked nuts, seeds, or dried fruit (wild figs, goji berries, raisins, dates) to take along with you.
- Experiment with new recipes weekly to keep interest and expand food choices.
- Make a blended salad (or green smoothie) when time is limited.
- Get sprouting! (See pages 44-45.)

Fats, protein, and starch put strain on the digestive system and require extra energy.

---

1. E₃Live is a nutritious, whole blue-green algae liquid that contains over sixty nutrients (including protein, essential fatty acids, and chlorophyll) that are 97 percent absorbable by the body. It is higher in chlorophyll content than wheatgrass and can help detoxify the body.

Shopping list

The following is a list of food options to start incorporating into your diet. You do not need to rush out and buy all of this right away! If you prefer to keep it simple and do without the nuts, dehydrated crackers, oils, salt, and sweeteners, you'll have better cleansing results. The simpler your meals, the deeper your cleanse. Just make sure to always have a variety of leafy greens in the fridge to make smoothies and simple salads.

Pre-cleanse week essentials (available for purchase at many health food stores):

- organic leafy greens, such as romaine, spinach, kale, collards, chard, parsley
- mixed organic greens
- sprouts (sunflower, buckwheat, pea, alfalfa, lentil, mung)
- wheatgrass juice (available fresh or frozen at various natural food stores)
- E₃Live (available in the freezer section of your natural food store) or other concentrated green food such as Vitamineral™ Green, chlorella, spirulina, barley grass, or Schinoussa Sea Vegetables™.
- lemons

Pre-cleanse week optional items (available at many health food stores):

- raw goodies (dehydrated crackers, high-quality raw energy bars)

For Gentle Option, week one:

- sweet potatoes or yams
- Manna bread (a frozen sprouted-grain bread)
- Ezekiel sprouted bread (a frozen sprouted-grain bread)
- millet, amaranth, or quinoa
- herbal teas (see page 113 for suggestions)

Raw staples (used in many recipes throughout the month-long program and available at many health food stores):

- purified water: if you don't have a filter at home, you can purchase reverse osmosis, spring, or distilled water, available in large refillable containers
- cold-pressed extra-virgin olive oil, flax or hemp oil, or Udo's Choice Oil Blend
- coconut oil (optional)
- unpasteurized apple cider vinegar
- raw agave or stevia[2] (sweeteners)
- dulse (a sea vegetable, excellent salt substitute, high in trace elements)
- nori (a sea vegetable used to make raw vegan sushi)
- unpasteurized miso (a soy product, good for seasoning)
- Nama Shoyu (raw soy sauce)
- raw olives[3]
- living sauerkraut

Add the following to your weekly grocery list:

- dark leafy greens of any kind (kale, romaine, spinach, collard, chard, arugula)
- cabbage (for Rejuvelac)
- fresh ripe fruit (apples, pears, lemons, bananas, persimmon)
- frozen fruit (freeze your own bananas, strawberries, mangos for smoothies and iced desserts)
- celery, avocados, cucumber, garlic, carrots, zucchini, tomatoes
- dried fruits (raisins, dates, figs, goji berries)
- nuts, seeds, and butters (in moderate amounts)
- raw almonds (soak for nut milks, snacking)
- raw hulled sunflower seeds (soak for pâté)
- raw un-hulled sunflower seeds (for sprouting, pâté)
- hemp seeds (smoothies, salads, sauces)
- flax seeds, chia seeds
- raw almond butter
- raw tahini
- grains and legumes (for sprouting during weeks two to four)
- rye berries, wheatberries, or quinoa
- lentils, peas, mung beans
- recommended supplemental foods (optional)
- full-spectrum plant-based enzymes
- raw maca (optional)
- bee pollen

2. Agave is a sweetener derived from the plant of the same name, usually available as a syrup. Stevia is a complex carbohydrate, valuable for those with hypoglycemia. It has a zero rating on the glycemic index and is a natural sweetener.

3. Sun-dried, raw olives are a good source of natural oils and minerals such as calcium. Please note that most olives are preserved with salt, packed in vinegar, and, if canned, heated during the canning process.

The following equipment will make your program easier:

- cutting board
- eight-inch chef's knife
- vegetable peeler
- blender (essential for smoothies, energy soup, dressings, nut milks)
- food processor (for pâté, chunkier sauces)
- juicer (for wheatgrass and greens)
- salad spinner
- spiral slicer (to prepare zucchini noodles)
- sprouting lids
- nut milk bag
- Mason jar for growing sprouts
- natural bristle dry skin brush
- tongue scraper
- enema bag

Breakfast

The easiest way to transition to the raw lifestyle is to begin with raw mornings. The morning hours are when the body is in its most active cleansing phase, so it is important to consume light, easy-to-digest foods such as fruits. Most fruits (with exceptions such as avocados, bananas, olives, and dried fruits) consist of 80 percent water. Eating high-water-content fruits during the morning hours allows the cleansing process to continue as fruits require very little energy to digest. Fruits—except for the more concentrated fruits listed above—pass through the digestive system quickly (about thirty minutes) without burdening the body's precious energy.

For optimal digestion, fruit is best eaten alone, on an empty stomach. Begin by eating juicier fruits such as oranges, grapefruits, apples, pears, peaches, and berries, leaving out dried fruits as they are more concentrated and slow down digestion. Find the amount that works for you and be aware that this might vary from day to day, especially when first transitioning. To place even less burden on the digestive system, try eating mono fruit meals, which means consuming one fruit at a time until satiation. This is an excellent method of accelerating the cleansing process.

Chewing plays an important role in healthy digestion, so be sure to chew each bite thoroughly, to a creamy consistency. Bananas take longer to digest, so save them for later in the morning when you are hungry and want a heavier food.

People with candida or other health conditions should consume green smoothies (without fruit) or freshly pressed green juice in the morning. These alkalizing drinks are easily assimilated by the body and require very little digestive energy.

Lunch

Once you feel comfortable with eating exclusively raw in the mornings, start including all raw lunches, focusing on high-water-content foods such as sprouts, fresh leafy greens, and raw vegetables. This will make two-thirds of your meals raw. There are endless ways to incorporate healthy raw lunches into your schedule. If you go to work every day, make sure to carry a large green smoothie or juice, a few pieces of fruit, soaked almonds, and goji berries in your lunch box. It's better to pack extra than not enough. Raw pâté, a dip, guacamole, veggie sticks, dehydrated crackers, and marinated kale salad keep well and are easily transported to the office.

If you go out for lunch with your colleagues, never leave on an empty stomach as you will be setting yourself up for temptation. Having a green smoothie, some nuts, a banana, avocado, or chia seeds will quickly curb your appetite. When lunching out, be sure to bring extras such as sunflower seeds, raisins, hemp seeds, or avocado to jazz up your salad. Bring your own homemade salad dressing.

Dinner

Dinner is usually the time to sit down with family to share not only a meal, but what's going on in our daily lives. It is an opportunity to talk about our day, enjoy a healthy meal together, and unwind. Regular family meals have been known to improve children's mental and physical health. It is an important time for parents to provide healthy role modeling for our children, a time everyone in the family looks forward to. If you find preparing meals rushed or stressful, enlist a helper from the family for meal preparation, such as washing and spin-drying lettuce, scrubbing carrots, and blending the soup or smoothies. Young children love getting involved, so teach them how to set the table or shred vegetables—and let them feel good about helping out!

For dinner meals, a large mixed salad, a raw veggie wrap, or zucchini "noodles" with an uncooked marinara sauce can be delicious for all family members to enjoy together. If you're still eating cooked foods, a small side dish of lightly steamed vegetables or cooked millet can be added to your raw meal.

Preparing both cooked and raw meals for you and your family can be time-consuming.

It requires patience, perseverance, and creativity, but it can be done! Time savers can include pre-washed organic salad greens, baby carrots, and cherry tomatoes, as well as preblended marinara sauce, soups, and pâtés. Double your favorite recipes and use them in different dishes. For example, a pâté can be used as a dip one night, then wrapped in collard leaves or stuffed in sushi rolls for the following night's dinner.

Explore new tastes!

Don't be afraid to experiment with food. Eating raw is about being creative and adventurous. Try out new raw fruits and vegetables as much as possible, and when you have time, test new recipes to expand your repertoire of favorite dishes. Detoxifying doesn't have to be all about sacrifices—focus on the new and tasty foods that you're including rather than those you are removing. There are so many mouth-watering new foods to discover. Relax, have fun with your food, and explore the endless variety!

A week before starting the program:

- Gradually reduce all caffeinated beverages to avoid withdrawal headaches.
- Cut back on all meat (including chicken and fish).
- Reduce all dairy products.
- Eliminate all sugar and white flour.
- Remove cooked temptations (foods not included on this program) from your kitchen.
- If you live with others, keep a separate detox cupboard for yourself.
- Plan your meals for a few days at a time before going shopping.
- Purchase enough fresh produce and supplies for the first few days of the program.
- Purchase enough purified drinking water for the first week of the program.
- Reschedule any potentially stressful or problematic events or activities that might occur during the program. This might include social outings with friends.
- For extra support, encourage a friend or adult family member to join you in your detox program.
- If you are a smoker, reduce the number of cigarettes each day and quit smoking before the beginning of the detox.

Coming off coffee

Caffeine is a powerful drug that affects the body's nervous system, brain, metabolism, blood pressure, heart rate, and gastrointestinal system. Because it overstimulates the adrenal glands, caffeine puts the body in a state of chronic stress. It also acts like a diuretic and can cause the body to lose calcium, which can lead to dehydration and bone loss over time, increasing the risk of developing osteoporosis. Since it stimulates the nervous system, excessive consumption of caffeine can also create problems such as anxiety, hypertension, muscle twitching, irritability, insomnia, heart palpitations, and sleep disorders.

Caffeine can be found in beverages such as coffee, black and green tea, chocolate, soft drinks, energy drinks, cold remedies, and pain medication. It is widely used throughout the world to provide a daily boost of energy or a heightened feeling of alertness. Coffee is highly addictive and can produce adverse withdrawal symptoms, such as headaches, fatigue, depression, anxiety, irritability, fatigue, and inability to concentrate, which can make quitting very challenging. Regular coffee drinkers often develop an increased tolerance, requiring even more caffeine to feed the addiction, which begins a further cycle of dependency.

When quitting coffee, remember you are withdrawing from a drug, so as the body detoxifies itself, be aware of withdrawal symptoms. The more caffeine you use, the worse withdrawal symptoms will be. Negative side effects generally last between one to three days, so stick with it, and you'll soon feel like a whole new person!

Tapering off gradually is easier for most people as an abrupt decrease can shock the body, causing severe withdrawal symptoms.

The following tips will help you ease off coffee:

- Dilute your coffee with water by half for a few days.
- Reduce daily cups of coffee by half.
- Slowly decrease to full decaf (use Swiss Water Process decaf only).
- Substitute decaf coffee with healthier grain coffees found at natural food stores.
- Replace coffee or decaf with herbal teas.
- Drink plenty of water.
- Alkalize the body with chlorophyll-rich foods.
- Have plenty of healthy convenient foods (apple slices, celery sticks, cucumbers) on hand, as you may need to snack more frequently throughout the day.
- Practice yoga.
- Get plenty of exercise.
- Avoid places you associate with drinking coffee.

As a former heavy espresso drinker, I found that E$_3$Live helped give me the brain boost that caffeine provided, but without the jitters. It also alkalized my body and lessened cravings. Instead of reaching for a coffee, I would drink an ounce or two of E$_3$Live whenever I needed. I also frequented the local juice bar and stood in line for my wheatgrass instead of waiting in the regular queue at Starbucks. Deep breathing, sweating, running, and exercising also helped me get off coffee, as these activities took me away from my mental/emotional clutter and into my physical body—and also got me in great shape!

The weekly schedule

The weekly schedule is an overview of the twenty-eight-day program. Each week corresponds to a different part of the program in which you make a gradual transition to a deeper cleanse. Use this schedule to track your progress.

DAY 1	DAY 2	DAY 3	DAY 4	DAY 5	DAY 6	DAY 7
Pre-cleanse Week 100% Vegan, 80%+ Raw						
← lasts all week →						

DAY 8	DAY 9	DAY 10	DAY 11	DAY 12	DAY 13	DAY 14
Week 2 100% Raw Vegan						
← lasts all week →						

DAY 15	DAY 16	DAY 17	DAY 18	DAY 19	DAY 20	DAY 21
Week 3 100% Living Foods	(Reduce concentrated foods by 50%)					
← lasts all week →						

DAY 22	DAY 23	DAY 24	DAY 25	DAY 26	DAY 27	DAY 28
Week 4 100% Living Foods	(No oils or concentrated foods)		Blended Foods		100% Living Foods (No oils or concentrated foods)	
← lasts 2 days →		← lasts 3 days →			← lasts 2 days →	

* Not everyone is prepared—physically, emotionally, or mentally—to jump into the detox program and complete the more intense weeks. Some of you may be coming from a lifetime of poor eating habits and may need to transition slower, remaining at week one or two for the duration of the program. On the other hand, many raw foodists will be ready to venture directly into week two or three. In other words, you may progress as slowly or as rapidly as you wish. As long as you are incorporating the principles in this book and commit to the SimplyRaw Detox Program for 28 days, you will not only achieve a great cleanse but you'll look and feel better than you ever dreamed possible!

Progress chart

Many people find it useful to keep track of their progress throughout the program. You can use the simple progress chart in this book, keep your own diary or blog, or use another method for keeping track of your journey. Recording your challenges, triumphs, feelings, emotions, and progress is a great way to release and share your journey. It also gives you an opportunity to reflect back on your experiences throughout the twenty-eight days to help keep you motivated.

DATE	WEIGHT	DETOX SYMPTOMS	POSITIVE CHANGES	CHALLENGES
Example: Oct. 8 First day of my detox!	**Example:** 125 lbs.	**Example:** Today ended with a slight headache (caffeine detox?) and fatigue. According to my husband, I was also a wee bit cranky. ☹	**Example:** I didn't give in to that Starbucks soy latte. Instead, I headed over to the juice bar for a shot of wheatgrass. It feels good to be making healthier food choices.	**Example:** I need to plan meals more in advance and have a decent supply of detox-friendly food within my reach! Going out for dinner with the gang and feeling the pressure was definitely a test!

WEEK-BY-WEEK MEAL PLANNER

Week 1 (Pre-cleanse):
100 percent vegan, 80 percent raw

This week will help you ease into the SimplyRaw Living Foods Detox Program, both physically and emotionally. The focus is on being 100 percent vegan, starting each day with raw food and consuming at least 80 percent raw foods the rest of the day. Remember that what you leave out of your diet is as important as what you eat. This week, eliminate all refined sugar, meat, and dairy, and all cooked foods except for lightly steamed veggies, millet, quinoa, and amaranth. Increase the amount of fresh raw foods to at least 80 percent. For maximum benefits, aim for 100 percent raw, if possible. Add at least ten ounces of green smoothies or green juice (see recipes in Appendix 1) to your daily diet.

Steaming is the best method of cooking food. Lightly steaming minimizes the loss of vitamins, minerals, and enzymes from your food.

Having a little cooked food for dinner is recommended this week, as it allows social leeway for evenings out with friends. Additionally, most people have cravings at night. To assist with digestion, take plant-based digestive enzymes with your cooked meals and eat only one type of steamed vegetable with a large salad or green smoothie.

If you're consuming cooked food, you also need to consume enzymes!

The elimination of animal products from the body enhances detoxification; meat and dairy are not only acidic but overtax the body and require extra energy and enzymes to digest. By omitting refined sugar (cake, cookies, candy, baked goods), processed starches (bread, pasta, cereal), wheat, and gluten, you'll soon notice health improvements.

Sprouts are the most important food groups. They are a living food and excellent source of oxygen, alkaline minerals, enzymes, and chlorophyll. Always make them the centerpiece of your meal.

What to expect

Everyone's detox process is personal and unique; the same program can have totally different effects depending on previous diet and lifestyle. Some people might feel good right away, but most will feel tired, headachy, achy, and even irritable, especially if they are heavy coffee or sugar consumers. As your body adjusts to these cleansing and nourishing new foods, you may experience discomfort.

Toxins can be stored in layers, and when one layer is removed, another deeper layer can be uncovered. This deeper layer must also be removed. This can result in a continued cycle of on-and-off again, roller-coaster ride of cleansing. When the toxins have been removed we often feel great, and then, when the body cleanses deeper and removes some of the older debris, we can feel worse. This can be discouraging for some people, but if you persevere and work through it, the symptoms of discomfort will taper off and you'll start to reap the rewards. During the program, especially the first week, try to rest as much as possible, and make sure you drink enough fluids.

When undergoing uncomfortable symptoms, remind yourself that the cleansing reaction is temporary, and this too will pass!

✓ EAT:

- green smoothies, green juice
- fresh fruit
- sprouts
- salads (focus on dark leafy greens such as kale, collards, chard, romaine, parsley, spinach, dandelion)
- Energy Soup
- fermented foods (sauerkraut, etc.)
- soaked nuts and seeds (in moderation)
- nut milk, seed cheese (in moderation)
- avocados
- raw olives
- raw almond butter, raw tahini (in moderation)
- dehydrated crackers
- raw desserts (in moderation)
- Rejuvelac (optional)
- herbal teas (optional)
- Lemon Water (see recipe, page 118)
- Fire Water (see recipe, page 117)
- small amounts of Himalayan Salt[4]
- dulse or kelp
- cold-pressed olive oil, flax or hemp oil, or Udo's Choice Oil Blend
- unpasteurized apple cider vinegar
- unpasteurized miso
- raw agave, stevia, unpasteurized honey
- small amounts of millet, quinoa, or amaranth
- limited amounts of steamed vegetables, sweet potatoes, or yams

---

4. Himalayan salt contains trace minerals. However, all salts are inorganic substances that may be difficult for the body to assimilate. For optimal health use kelp and dulse instead.

HAVE EVERY DAY:

- water (half your body weight in ounces) to help remove toxins
- Lemon Water, Fire Water
- fresh green smoothies and/or green juice
- one to two ounces fresh wheatgrass juice
- one to two tablespoons concentrated greens[5], E$_3$Live, Vitamineral™ Greens, Schinoussa Sea Vegetables™, spirulina, and/or chlorella to provide nutritional support throughout the program

---

During a detox, old emotions are often brought to the surface and we may feel irritable, depressed, or cranky. Be prepared to work with these old emotions. Identify them, write in your journal, and let them go. Reward yourself with a massage or sauna.

✗ ELIMINATE:

- all meat including chicken, turkey, fish, seafood
- dairy products (including cheese, milk, yogurt, butter, feta)
- eggs (or foods containing eggs)
- refined sugar (chocolate, candy, cookies, gum)
- raw cacao[6]
- peanuts
- fried foods
- pasta, packaged cereals
- all cooked foods except for lightly steamed veggies, millet, quinoa, and amaranth
- soy products (soy milk, tofu)
- tamari and Braggs Liquid Aminos
- white flour and rice
- coffee and all tea[7] except for herbal teas
- pasteurized juices (including all canned, boxed, and bottled juices. Unless it is freshly pressed, do not consume.)
- alcohol[8] in all forms
- vinegars (except for unpasteurized apple cider vinegar)
- bread and yeast products (Ezekiel and Manna sprouted breads are acceptable during the first week)

---

5. Concentrated greens provide added vitamins and minerals and encourage healing on a daily basis.

6. Cacao is a stimulant containing caffeine, theobromine, and oxalic acid, which binds calcium. Cacao contains some saturated fat and is considered to be acid-forming in the body by some health experts. It can can dilate blood vessels, increase speed of heartbeat, and cause anxiety and headaches.

7. Coffee and tea are stimulants that can stress your adrenal glands and make your energy levels erratic. Many soft drinks have a similar effect and are also high in sugar, artificial additives, colors, and aspartame—all harmful to the body.

8. Alcohol has a high calorie content. It can also damage the liver.

When uncooked foods are included in a meal, always eat the raw foods first.

While Rejuvelac and Energy Soup are key components of the SimplyRaw Living Foods Detox Program, they are not mandatory. Make sure to drink green smoothies or juices if Energy Soup isn't possible, and if you can't drink Rejuvelac, be sure to consume some living sauerkraut and take probiotics[9] daily.

There is no portion control or calorie counting on the program. Pay attention to your body's signals and eat until satisfied without overeating. If you're adjusting from a heavy cooked-food diet or are physically active, you may need to eat more as you transition.

Sample day:

(See recipes in Appendix 1 for other options.)

There is no fixed daily menu for the program, as each individual requires different quantities of food depending on metabolic type, age, activity level, and many other factors. We encourage you to listen to your body, eating when physically hungry and stopping when satisfied. Observe your body for signs that you are comfortably full—not stuffed. Stop eating when you're halfway through your meal and ask yourself what your current fullness level is. Pay attention to your body. Do not overeat!

Always bring your own! Don't risk setting yourself up for temptation when you leave home. Make sure to have food to nibble on, no matter where you go—running a quick errand, visiting friends, watching a movie, or going out for dinner. (Easy-access foods include apples, dried fruit, almonds, dulse, bee pollen, or a quick smoothie.)

9. Probiotics are living organisms found in our intestines. These friendly bacteria are important in maintaining the body's delicate balance of beneficial bacteria—an essential element to good digestive health and a strong immune system.

Upon rising:
1–2 oz wheatgrass juice or
1–2 tbsp E₃Live or concentrated greens and
Lemon Water (room temperature or warm) or Fire Water (see recipes section) or herbal tea

Breakfast:
Fresh ripe fruit and/or fruit smoothie or
green smoothie or green juice

Mid-morning:
ripe banana or
green smoothie or green juice (cucumber, celery, sprouts, parsley)

Noon:
mixed green salad with sprouts, half avocado, sauerkraut, and dulse
sprout salad with a slice of rye Manna bread and tomatoes or
green smoothie

Mid-afternoon:
small handful of soaked almonds or goji berries or
green juice and/or 1–2 oz wheatgrass

Dinner:
Energy Soup and seed cheese and veggie sticks or
large salad with Italian pâté
Gentle Option: large sprout salad with either millet or steamed
vegetable with 1 tbsp cold-pressed oil

Evening snack:
sliced apple with dulse or
nut milk shake or
herbal tea

---

*Millet, quinoa and amaranth are all gluten-free grains.
*Manna bread and Ezekial bread are not raw but sprouted and easier to digest.
*Nuts and seeds become more digestible and increase in nutritional value when germinated by soaking in purified water overnight. After draining, they can be stored in the refrigerator for up to five days. Soaked nuts and seeds are handy to have available for making milks, pâtés, or just snacking on—in moderation, of course.

If you feel that the program is too intense and you need to eat something more substantial, one cup of lightly steamed vegetables (cauliflower, broccoli, yams, or sweet potatoes) is acceptable. However, for best results, follow the weekly suggestions.

Week 2: 100 percent raw vegan

This week continues the transition toward living foods, while introducing you to a broad range of raw vegan options. Any raw vegan foods can be eaten this week (including dehydrated crackers, pâtés, soaked nuts and seeds, nut and seed cheeses, almond butter, and some desserts) but as side dishes. Do not overeat these concentrated foods as they are hard to digest and slow down the detoxification process. Sprouts and leafy greens are a large component of the program. Drink at least one quart of green smoothies or green juice every day, and have a large sprout salad or Energy Soup with lunch and dinner. Continue eating ripe fruit in the morning (unless you have candida), and enjoy the abundance of raw plant foods. Incorporate enemas daily and colonics once during this period (see pages 95 and 97).

If you haven't already, take a moment to write down your reasons for cleansing and what you want for yourself. Be very specific. Outlining your goals from the beginning will keep you motivated and strong.

Raw and living foods are cleansing, rejuvenating, and energizing. They are loaded with the vital nutrients necessary for producing healthy cells and include the fiber necessary for regular bowel movements. They are also excellent in bringing more of an acid-alkaline balance to the body while nourishing it with an abundance of enzymes, oxygen, vitamins, minerals, and antioxidants.

Eating raw means no cooking. All fruits and vegetables are eaten raw, while nuts, seeds, and grains are soaked or sprouted for optimal digestion.

✓ EAT:

- green smoothies
- a large serving of sprouts with every meal (or as your meal)
- Energy Soup or other blended soups
- fresh green juices (sprouts, celery, cucumber, kale)
- fruit smoothies
- Rejuvelac (optional)
- nut and seed cheeses
- nut milks (in small amounts as these are concentrated foods and will slow down the cleansing process)
- fresh fruits and fresh vegetables, such as dark leafy greens such as kale, spinach, collards, chard, dandelion, arugula, parsley, cilantro
- soaked nuts and seeds (in moderation)
- sauerkraut
- sprouted grains and legumes such as buckwheat, quinoa, and lentils.
- dulse (for seasoning)
- Nama Shoyu (in moderation)
- small amounts of Himalayan salt
- unpasteurized miso (small amounts)
- herbal teas (optional)
- steamed veggies (for Gentle Option)

Eat anything you want—as long as it's raw and vegan. The focus, however, is always on sprouts and leafy greens. If you wish, herbal teas are allowed.

CONTINUE DAILY:

- Drink purified water (half your body weight in ounces).
- Drink one quart of green smoothies.
- Have two tablespoons concentrated greens.
- Drink one to two ounces wheatgrass juice.

✗ ELIMINATE (IN ADDITION TO LAST WEEK'S SUGGESTIONS):

- all cooked food including grains
- Manna and Ezekial breads

Fruits are excellent for cleansing, while greens help build and restore the body's nutrient needs.

Sample day:

(See recipes in Appendix 1 for more options.)

Remember to always honor your hunger and eat only when physically hungry. Any foods (healthy or not) eaten beyond the body's need are a burden. If you have any doubts whether you are really hungry or not, you probably aren't! True hunger is unmistakable. (Try drinking a large glass of water instead.)

Upon rising:
1–2 oz wheatgrass juice or
2 or more tbsp E3Live (followed with water) or
concentrated greens and
Lemon Water or Fire Water or herbal tea

Breakfast:
fruit smoothie and/or fresh fruit or
green smoothie or green juice

Drink water and/or Rejuvelac between meals.

Mid-morning:
1 apple and/or
6–8 soaked almonds

Lunch:
green smoothie or green juice or
mixed green salad and guacamole or
Collard Roll-ups filled with Sunflower Pâté and sprouts (see recipes in
Appendix 1)

Pay attention to how your body feels.

Mid-afternoon:
1-2 oz wheatgrass juice or
2 tbsp concentrated greens and green juice or
nut milk shake

Dinner:
Energy Soup and nut or seed cheese or
Quick and Easy Spinach-Apple Soup with dehydrated crackers or
Marinated Kale Salad with Sunflower Pâté and veggie sticks or
Zucchini Noodles with Pesto Sauce (see recipes in Appendix 1)

Gentle Option:
Large salad with a side dish of lightly steamed vegetables and 1 tbsp
cold-pressed oil

Evening snack:
Frozen Vanilla Bliss (see recipe in Appendix 1) or
1 apple with dulse or
herbal tea

As soon as you eat cooked foods, the detoxification process is reduced. Stick
with the program. Your body will thank you for it! Visualize all the positive
effects you wish to experience from your detox.

As you cleanse your body, you may notice changes with your taste buds. Initially,
green smoothies or Energy Soup may not be as palatable as they will become during
the detox program. Your taste buds have become desensitized from eating processed
foods and excess salt, sugar, oil, and spices. Within a week or so after you begin
cleansing your body of toxins, your taste buds readapt, and you can begin to enjoy
consuming these foods.

When cravings arise:

- Remind yourself that cravings are usually short-term and will pass.
- Think of the consequences of giving in to your cravings.
- If you're tired, take a nap.
- Read a good book.
- Drink water.
- Be kind to yourself.
- Take a warm bath with essential oils.
- Rebound, jump, skip!
- Drink a shooter of E₃Live.
- Drink a green smoothie or juice.
- Eat something raw.
- Nurture what's really missing in your life.
- Visit with a friend.
- Reconnect with your loved one.
- Take a walk or hike.
- Get a hug!
- Breathe deeply.

Fill out your Progress Chart.

Week 3: 100 percent living foods

"Energy Soup is the most important nourishment in the Living Foods Lifestyle." —Ann Wigmore

This week, focus on fresh, easy-to-digest, 100 percent living nutrition such as sprouts, dark leafy greens, and other chlorophyll-rich foods. Drink one quart of green smoothies or juice each day, and if you haven't already, consume Rejuvelac and Energy Soup regularly. Be sure to eat plenty of sprouts (sunflower, buckwheat, pea, alfalfa, clover, and broccoli), and drink two to three ounces of fresh wheatgrass juice and E₃Live daily.

Both raw and living foods contain enzymes; however, the enzyme and oxygen content in livings foods is much higher. These foods are made easier to digest through soaking, sprouting, and fermenting. Sprouts provide up to thirty times more nutrition than the best organic vegetables and fruits!

Living foods are packed with the enzymes, chlorophyll, and oxygen needed to fuel our cells. They allow the body to focus its resources on cleansing and rebuilding the immune system. These foods include nutritious, power-packed sprouts, fermented foods, nut and seed cheeses, Rejuvelac, Energy Soup, Flax Cream, soaked nuts and seeds, and wheatgrass juice. They are easily digested and leave you energized, rather than tired, after meals.

Raw antioxidants help slow free-radical damage to cells and tissues.

✓ CONTINUE TO EAT DAILY:

- water (half your body weight in ounces)
- green smoothies and green juices
- Energy Soup
- two to three ounces of wheatgrass juice
- two or more tablespoons concentrated greens (E$_3$Live, Vitamineral™ Green, Schinoussa Sea Vegetables™, chlorella, blue-green algae)

INCORPORATE:

- enemas daily and colonics once during this period (see pages 96 and 98).

✗ ELIMINATE (IN ADDITION TO LAST WEEK'S SUGGESTIONS):

- almond butter, tahini
- sprouted grains (except for Rejuvelac)
- corn
- all extracted sweeteners (honey, maple syrup, agave)
- all salt (substitute dulse or kelp for seasoning)
- Nama Shoyu sauce
- all vinegar (substitute lemon juice)
- olives

✗ REDUCE BY 50 PERCENT (FOR BEST DETOX RESULTS, ELIMINATE COMPLETELY):

- oils (see recipes for oil-free salad dressings)
- concentrated foods such as soaked nuts, seeds, desserts, crackers, dried fruits, bars (seed cheeses, Flax Cream, and Chia Cream are acceptable in moderation)
- nut and seed milks

You are what you eat—or rather, assimilate. This old saying has a lot of validity: Dietary choices are the cornerstone to good health and can produce incredible results to balance overall well-being. To ensure that you are assimilating your meals, always be sure to chew, chew, chew (yes, even blended foods).

Sample day:

(See recipes in Appendix 1 for more options)

Upon rising:
wheatgrass juice, E₃Live or other concentrated greens and
Lemon Water or Fire Water or herbal tea

Breakfast:
fresh fruit or green smoothie or green juice

Mid-morning:
ripe papaya or Green Banana Pudding (see recipe in Appendix 1)

Lunch:
Energy Soup with 2 tbsp seed cheese or
Sprout Salad with seed cheese, sauerkraut, and nori

Mid-afternoon:
1–2 tbsp wheatgrass or concentrated greens and
green smoothie or green juice

Dinner:
Energy Soup or Wigmore's Health Salad with Sauerkraut and
Red Peppers stuffed with sprouts and Guacamole (see recipes in
Appendix 1)
Gentle Option: large sprout salad with lightly steamed (mono)
veggies

Evening snack:
Banana Mango Spinach Pudding or Carob Milk (see recipes in
Appendix 1) or
1 apple with dulse

Reflect on your personal goals and motivation.

If your cleansing reactions are severe, you may be detoxifying too rapidly. Cut back on the program and try these suggestions:.

- Drink extra pure water, fresh juices, herbal teas and/or smoothies to help flush out toxins.
- Take plenty of deep breaths.
- Have an enema or colonic (see pages 95 and 97).
- Take a brisk walk in the fresh air.
- Practice yoga.
- Do mild exercises, such as rebounding.
- Splurge on a massage.
- Get light sun exposure.
- Take a brief nap or rest break.
- Dry skin brush.
- Soak in the tub.

- Take an infrared sauna to sweat out more toxins.
- Use peppermint essential oil for headaches, stomach aches, or other symptoms that may arise.
- Use positive affirmations. Tell yourself that your body is eliminating harmful toxins and you are becoming cleaner and healthier with every day.
- Write in your journal.

Week 4 (Days 1, 2): 100 percent living foods—no oils or concentrated foods

This week is essentially the same as the second week, but you will be eliminating all nuts and seeds (except for Flax or Chia Cream), oils, and dehydrated foods. Consume green smoothies and juices, and one blended soup daily, preferably Energy Soup. Focus on chlorophyll- and oxygen-rich foods such as sprouts and dark leafy greens. Drink wheatgrass juice and Rejuvelac.

To get your essential fatty acids, make sure to include two to four tablespoons of Flax or Chia Cream in green smoothies and Energy Soup.

✓ EAT (IN ORDER OF IMPORTANCE TO THE DETOX):

- Energy Soup
- sprouts
- wheatgrass juice, E$_3$Live, concentrated greens
- green smoothies, green juices
- salads
- blended soups
- avocado (no more than half per day)
- ripe fruit
- fruit smoothies
- dulse or kelp
- Rejuvelac (recommended)
- Lemon Water, herbal teas
- lightly steamed veggies for Gentle Option

Mineral-rich, nutrient-dense foods are nature's true fountain of youth.

CONTINUE DAILY:

- Drink plenty of purified water (half your body weight in ounces).
- Eat Energy Soup.
- Drink green smoothies and green juices.
- Two tablespoons or more concentrated greens.
- Drink two to three ounces of wheatgrass juice.
- Take enemas.

✗ ELIMINATE:

- all oils
- nut milks
- dehydrated foods
- all energy bars
- dried fruits
- nuts and seeds

INCORPORATE:

- one colonic

Substitute avocado for oil in salad dressings, but don't overdo it!

Sample day:

 Upon rising:
1–2 oz wheatgrass juice or
2 or more tbsp E₃Live or other concentrated green and
Lemon Water or Fire Water or herbal tea

Breakfast:
fruit or fruit smoothie or
green smoothie or green juice

Mid-morning:
Berry Smoothie or Mangocado Pudding (see recipes in Appendix 1)

 Lunch:
green smoothie or
Kale Salad (no oil) with sprouts or
Creamy Kale Soup (see recipes in Appendix 1)

Mid-afternoon:
1–2 oz wheatgrass or
2 or more tbsp concentrated greens and
sliced apples or pears

 Dinner:
a. Energy Soup with Flax Cream or avocado and It's a Wrap or
b. Sprout Salad with Nori Rolls (see recipes in Appendix 1)
Gentle Option:
Any of the above with 1 cup of lightly steamed mono-veggies

Evening snack:
Pineapple-Banana Drink or
Papaya Pudding (see recipes in Appendix 1) or
herbal teas

Stay positive

It is important to remain as positive as you can throughout the program. This is an exciting adventure. Believe in your detox journey and stick with it confidently.

Remember, the mind runs the body. If you can't do the program 100 percent, do the best you can. Try not to get down on yourself—emotional toxins can be much worse than a few bites of something not-so-healthy!

The most important thing is to consume a large amount of live, chlorophyll-rich foods. Focus on creating health, and be patient with the process. Believe in yourself. Acknowledge the positive changes and the progress you're making to improve your health and quality of life. Be gentle and loving with yourself.

Week 4 (Days 3, 4, 5): Three days of blending

For the following three days, focus on easy-to-digest nourishment such as Energy Soup, green drinks, green smoothies, blended soups, and simple puddings. For best results, eat Energy Soup at least once a day.

Raw, dark leafy greens are extremely nutritious but can be difficult to digest because of their tough outer cell wall. These cells (cellulose) need to be ruptured in order to assimilate the vital nutrients within the tough outer structures. This is made possible by chewing to a creamy consistency or by blending.

Blending is an excellent way to obtain nutrients in an easy-to-digest form. It can make a dramatic improvement to our health. Without stressing the digestive system, we save energy, thus allowing the body to eliminate waste and focus on self-healing. During this period, it is especially important to help with the elimination process through dry skin brushing, enemas, colonics, and/or saunas. (See more on complementary detox therapies, pages 92–99.)

For best results, eat blended foods in small amounts throughout the day. Your stomach does not have teeth, so remember to chew your food thoroughly! This includes chewing all liquids and blended foods.

Drinking fresh juices and green smoothies are an easy way to get more vitamins and minerals into your body.

Energy Soup is not only nourishing and detoxifying, but the fiber content also helps to clean the intestines and digestive system. The more Energy Soup you eat, the better you will cleanse. Two to four tablespoons of Flax or Chia Cream can be added to green smoothies or as a topping to your bowl of Energy Soup, provided that you don't use avocados. Seed cheese can also be eaten in moderation—but consume only one fat per meal.

If you've been following the Gentle Option with lightly steamed veggies, try going all the way, eating only blended foods for the next three days.

✓ EAT:

- wheatgrass juice, E₃Live, Vitamineral™ Greens, Schinoussa Sea Vegetables™, or other concentrated greens
- Energy Soup at least once per day
- green smoothies, green juice
- fruit smoothies, blended fruit, in moderation
- blended soups without oil
- seed cheeses (small amount with soups)
- Flax Cream (small amount with Energy Soup or smoothies)
- chia seeds, soaked (small amount, blended in smoothies or soups)
- Rejuvelac
- dulse, kelp (as seasoning), blended in Energy Soup
- Lemon Water, Fire Water
- herbal teas (optional)

Energy Soup for energy!

✗ ELIMINATE:

- all solid food
- salt
- sweeteners
- dried fruits

Juice your food and chew your juice!

CONTINUE DAILY:

- plenty of purified water throughout the day (half your body weight in ounces)
- wheatgrass juice or E₃Live (or other concentrated greens)
- Energy Soup
- one quart of green smoothie or juice
- dry skin brushing
- tongue scraping
- light exercise
- enemas

Sample day:

(See recipes in Appendix 1 for more options.)

 Upon rising:
wheatgrass juice, E₃Live, or other concentrated greens and
Lemon Water or Fire Water or
herbal tea

Breakfast:
fruit smoothie or green smoothie or green juice

Mid-morning:
green juice or
Banana Milk (see recipe in Appendix 1)

 Lunch:
green smoothie with Flax Cream or
Energy Soup with Flax Cream or
Spinach Soup and Seed Cheese (see recipes in Appendix 1)

Mid-afternoon:
wheatgrass juice or concentrated greens and/or
green juice

Dinner:
Energy Soup with Flax Cream or
Cool Cucumber Soup with seed cheese

Evening snack:
Living Papaya Pudding or
Banana Milk or herbal tea

Coping with hunger

Here are a few suggestions to help you deal with hunger (whether physical or emotional):

- Sip Lemon Water, Rejuvelac, Fire Water, herb teas, fresh diluted green juice, a smoothie, or plain water.
- Focus on the feeling. Often our experience of hunger is an emotional one and linked to feelings of grief, anger, guilt, pleasure, love, etc.
- Move your body. Stretch. Go for a walk. Take a hike. Hit the yoga mat. Rebound.
- Listen to some good tunes and dance like no one's watching!
- Talk to a friend.
- Play a game with your family.
- Write in your journal.

- Read an absorbing book.
- Hand-write a letter to a friend.
- Start a photo album, scrap book, or knitting project.
- Watch a movie.
- Soak in the tub with natural oils and candles.
- Treat yourself to a massage, facial, manicure, or far-infrared sauna.

- Meditate.
- Unclutter closets, drawers, and shelves.
- Clean the fridge.
- Organize your office.
- Sort through unused clothes and give them away.
- Book a colonic.
- Go for a run.
- Breathe!

Week 4 (Days 6, 7): 100 percent living foods—no oils or concentrated foods

Easing back to solid foods takes time and discipline. Do not overdo it, otherwise you'll overtax the body and defeat the purpose of your detox. Continue to eat blended foods as much as possible while incorporating quick-transit, high-water solids such as fruit, fresh salads, sprouts, and leafy greens. Remember to always chew food well so that it is more easily digested. Make sure to wait at least two days after the end of week four before eating soaked nuts or other concentrated foods (and then consume in moderation), as they are very difficult on the digestive system and can stress the body. A few tablespoons of seed cheese is fine as it has been fermented and is easier to digest. Do not rush this process. Pay attention to how your body feels. If you experience bloating, gurgling, or gas, take this as a sign to slow down and eat smaller meals.

Once you have completed the program and reintroduced more foods into your diet, pay attention to your body, and look for changes in energy levels, digestion, cravings, bloating, and other such symptoms. Follow a varied diet based on the key foods in this manual (fresh, uncooked fruits and vegetables with an emphasis on sprouts, leafy greens, Energy Soup, green smoothies, juice, fermented foods) to sustain your health and well-being.

Keep your meals simple.

✓ EAT:

- green smoothies, green juices
- fruit smoothies
- sprouts
- Energy Soup
- Flax Cream (with Energy Soup)
- blended soups
- salads
- fresh ripe fruit
- avocados, in moderation
- seed cheese, in moderation
- dulse or kelp
- Rejuvelac

✗ AVOID FOR THE NEXT TWO DAYS:

- nuts, seeds, nut and seed milks, nut and seed butters
- dehydrated foods
- sprouted grains
- salt
- sweeteners
- dried fruits
- oils
- all sweeteners (except for stevia)

Appreciate the new and improved health your body radiates!

Sample day:

(See recipes in Appendix 1 for more options.)

 Upon rising:
1–2 oz wheatgrass juice or
E₃Live or other concentrated green and
Lemon Water or Fire Water or herbal tea

Breakfast:
Fresh melon or other fruit or
green smoothie or green juice

Mid-morning:
Berry Smoothie or
Mangocado Pudding

 Lunch:
Energy Soup and seed cheese or
Kale Salad with sprouts

Afternoon snack:
1–2 oz wheatgrass and/or
green juice or green smoothie

Dinner:
Garden Salad with sprouts and/or
Nori Rolls with avocado, cucumber, and sprouts

Evening snack:
Flax-ative (see recipe in Appendix 1) or
herbal tea

Reflect on your four-week journey.

Complementary detox therapies

Our bodies' systems are intricately designed to self-cleanse; however, additional supportive therapies can be introduced to enhance the body's response to the detox. The therapies listed below not only complement the detox program by assisting with the elimination of toxins, they also help the body to adjust to these changes. Additionally, these rituals will help you feel and look your best! Complementary detoxification approaches help support your detox program.

Dry skin brushing

"Daily dry skin brushing increases the activity of pores and eliminates more waste materials (uric acid crystals, catarrh and impurities) than any soap and water." —Ann Wigmore Institute

The skin, sometimes called the third kidney because of its eliminative function, is the largest organ of your body. It is responsible for one quarter of the body's detoxification, making it one of the most important eliminative organs. When you dry skin brush, you help your lymph system cleanse itself of toxins that collect in the lymph glands. It helps the detoxification process by increasing circulation, stimulating the lymphatic system, opening the pores, and invigorating the skin.

Dry skin brushing removes the top dead layer of skin, encouraging new cells to rejuvenate. It helps make the skin glow. The gentle brushing of the bristles also has a beneficial effect on cellulite and is one of the easiest methods to improve your overall health and beauty.

There are various types of brushes, available at most health food stores. You will need a brush with a handle (some are detachable) so that you can reach all the inaccessible parts of your back. Make sure that your brush is a natural (not synthetic) bristle brush, so it won't scratch the surface of the skin.

If you don't have a dry skin brush, a loofah may also be used as long as it isn't wet. If using a loofah, you'll need a softer brush, or a flannel, for your face.

Benefits of dry skin brushing:

- stimulates the lymphatic system
- helps eliminate toxins from the body
- increases circulation
- helps digestion
- strengthens immune system
- encourages cells to regenerate
- removes dead skin layers
- helps combat cellulite
- improves muscle tone
- stimulates the nervous system and brings a great sense of well-being
- invigorates and enhances your general health

Dry skin brush each part of your body daily, just before showering. Do not brush wet skin as it won't have the same effect. Always brush toward the heart, beginning from the soles of your feet.

How to brush:
1. With long sweeping strokes, work upward from the soles of your feet to the legs and thighs.
2. Move brush across your stomach and buttocks.
3. Sweep brush from the palm of your hand toward your elbow and shoulder.
4. Move from the neck down toward back and/or chest.

Tips:
- The best time to brush is before your shower, after your morning exercise, and before breakfast (on an empty stomach).
- Brush gently where the skin is thinnest (use a softer brush for your face).
- Always use a natural fiber brush.
- If your new brush is too rough, or you wish to clean it, wash it with water and mild soap and let it dry in the sun.
- The brush is personal—do not share it with anyone else.

Tongue scraping

A clean mouth is a healthy mouth. Scraping the tongue removes bacteria and toxic metabolic substances of the gut that are deposited on the tongue overnight. This coating is a waste product that should be cleaned away every morning, otherwise it will be ingested again when eating breakfast. Buildup of bacteria on the tongue causes bad breath (halitosis), and various types of digestive and respiratory problems can result from continued absorption of these waste products.

How to use a tongue scraper:
1. Stick out your tongue.
2. Take the tongue scraper in hand and reach toward the back of the tongue.
3. Scrape forward several times, rinsing the white mucus off the scraper between scrapings.
4. Rinse out your mouth once you are done.

Rebounding

Rebounding is a convenient and metabolically effective form of exercise performed in the comfort of your own home or office. The folding rebounder (or mini-trampoline) can travel along with you during trips.

The rebounding motion stimulates all internal organs, moves the cerebral-spinal fluid, and is beneficial for the intestines. It strengthens the immune system and is much easier on the joints than running on a conventional surface.

Health benefits of regular rebounding:

- increases lung capacity
- circulates more oxygen to the tissues
- aids lymphatic circulation as well as blood flow in the circulatory system
- helps prevent cardiovascular disease
- helps normalize blood pressure
- increases production of red blood cells
- strengthens the heart and other muscles in the body
- lowers elevated cholesterol and triglyceride levels
- improves digestion and elimination
- stimulates the metabolism, thereby reducing the likelihood of obesity
- burns calories and helps shape the legs without the impact of running
- tones up the glandular system, especially the thyroid
- encourages better relaxation and improved sleep
- relieves fatigue and menstrual discomfort for women
- improves healing processes
- minimizes the number of colds, allergies, and digestive disturbances by boosting the immune system
- improves mental performance
- helps combat depression
- offers a fun way to exercise

Epsom salt baths

For generations, Epsom salts have been used in baths to help reduce stress and alleviate aches and pains. It is also a simple way to draw toxins out of the body. When magnesium sulphate (Epsom salt) is absorbed through the skin in a hot bath, it stimulates lymph drainage and draws toxins out through the pores. It also helps reduce swelling and relaxes muscles.

One to two cups of Epsom salts (purchased from most health food stores and pharmacies) in a tub of hot water can help soothe nerves and restore a sense of well-being.

Lymphatic massage

Lymphatic massage or drainage is a gentle, rhythmic massage of points on the body where lymph nodes are located. It is used to relieve congestion in the lymphatic system. It improves circulation, reduces edema, and stimulates the immune system to eliminate toxins. Generally administered by a trained massage therapist, lymphatic massage can be relaxing and soothing to the body.

Far-infrared sauna

Unlike traditional high heat saunas, far-infrared saunas warm the body in the same manner as natural sunlight but without the harmful ultraviolet rays. These special saunas help expel harmful toxins from the body utilizing ceramic heaters that allow the heat to penetrate up to three inches into the tissues. Far-infrared saunas are a powerful means of cellular cleansing as they increase metabolism and blood circulation. In addition to their use for detoxification, they can also relax muscles and rejuvenate the body.

In her book *Detoxify or Die* (Prestige, 2002), Dr Sherry Rogers says an infrared sauna is the only way of removing man-made toxins from your body.

Deep breathing

Breathing is essential to life. We can go weeks without food and days without water, but only minutes without breathing. Oxygen is the most vital of all nutrients, yet most of us deprive ourselves of oxygen by not breathing deeply enough. Practicing deep breathing is an effective way of oxygenating our blood. It also helps remove toxins and waste products from our cells. Breathing deeply enhances the immune system and general state of health.

Colonic irrigation

A safe, gentle way to remove impacted mucus and waste from the colon, colonics, also known as colon hydrotherapy or colonic irrigation, promotes peristalsis of the intestines, hydrates the colon with pure water, and expels parasites. The practice dates back to Egyptian times. Colonic irrigation is similar to enemas, but involves larger amounts of water and is administered by a certified colon therapist. By repeatedly introducing and expelling water, in conjunction with gentle abdominal massage, impacted feces and toxins are softened, dissolved, and removed.

The colon is one of the body's five major organs of elimination and is often referred to as the body's sewer system. When you do not eliminate properly, feces deposits build up along the wall or in the pockets of the colon. When the bowels become toxic, the blood picks up these bowel toxins. Poor function of the colon may therefore contribute to headaches, fatigue, and sluggishness.

Maintaining regular elimination is crucial to overall health. Health experts and therapists such as Bernard Jensen, Norman Walker, Ann Wigmore, Richard Anderson, and Paavo Airola were all proponents of enemas and colonic irrigation and believed that constipation is the underlying root of many diseases and illnesses. Norman Walker, a nutritionist and researcher, called constipation "the number one affliction underlying nearly every ailment." He was an early advocate of fresh, raw vegetable juices, positive attitude, and regular colon cleansing as the way to feel young and healthy. He wrote, "There is no ailment, sickness or disease that will not respond to treatment quicker and more effectively than it will after the administration of a series of colon irrigations."

Today, laxatives have often replaced the use of both enemas and colonics. The large scale of laxative sales suggests that constipation is a major health condition for people eating a standard North American diet.

A series of colonics can enhance any cleansing regime. The number of sessions desired will depend on the individual. However, I recommend at least one colonic at the beginning of the program, one during the middle, and one at the end.

Regular cleansing of the colon helps rid the body of impacted fecal material, mucus, parasites, yeast, intestinal stress, and unwanted bacteria. Benefits include a reduction of toxins, improved peristalsis function and inner ecology, improved absorption of nutrients, healthier blood circulation, and a general feeling of well-being.

"The Most Important Part of the Body"

excerpted with permission from *Cleansing the Body and the Colon for a Happier, Healthier You Using Herbal Fiberblend* by Teresa Schumacher and Toni Schumacher Lund (Herbal Fiberblend, 1997)

One day the body parts got together and decided to have a board meeting. Here's what went on behind closed doors. There was intense discussion to determine who was the most important part of the body.

The BRAIN was the first to speak. "Without me, nothing would be accomplished."

Then the HEART spoke up. "Without me pumping blood to your brain, you could not function."

The ARMS laughed. "You're both wrong, without me to put food in the mouth, nothing would work."

The LEGS quickly added, "Without me you couldn't get your food."

The STOMACH said, "Without me, your food would not digest."

The LUNGS bellowed back, "Without me, you couldn't breathe."

The EYES blinked, "Without me you could not see."

The KIDNEYS snorted, "Without me, you could not detoxify and eliminate."

The COLON meekly spoke up. "I am important. You need me to eliminate all of the garbage from your systems."

Everyone laughed and made fun of him. "How can you be as important as we are? You're just a smelly old sewer." The poor colon ... his feelings were hurt. He turned away, and thought, I'll show them. He shut down! Then he sat back and watched what would happen.

The BRAIN was stupefied.
The HEART'S beat was weak.
The ARMS and LEGS were weak and couldn't move.
The LUNGS breathing was shallow.
The EYES became cloudy.
The KIDNEYS quit.

Then the COLON looked around and decided it was time to call another meeting. It wasn't too lively this time, but everyone was in total agreement: The colon was the most important organ in the body.

Enemas

Maintaining regular elimination is crucial to overall health. Enemas and colon cleansing play an important role in health by clearing the body of toxins and impacted waste. A clean colon leads to improved health. When the bowel is dirty, the blood is dirty, as are the organs and tissues. Therefore, the bowel must be cared for first, before any effective healing can take place.

Enemas are a safe, effective, and ancient remedy for all kinds of ailments. They efficiently clean the colon of fecal matter in the lower portion of the intestine and are an excellent remedy for relieving headaches, constipation, gas, colds, fever, backache, fecal concentration, and toxic buildup.

Although not required for the program, it is highly recommended to take one enema every day from the second week onward, and especially during the three days of blending. A series of at least three colonics throughout the program is also recommended. This will help free any blockages and help speed up toxin removal.

Enema bags, sometimes called "fountain syringes," can be found at most pharmacies or online. They look like a hot water bottle and come with a tube, an adjustable clamp, a nozzle, and a hook for hanging on the door or shower curtain.

HOW TO TAKE AN ENEMA

Equipment needed:

- enema bag
- castor, olive, or sesame oil as lubricant for enema tip
- purified or distilled water
- towel (for your head and for kneeling on)

1. Rinse bag and nozzle to ensure cleanliness.

2. Fill enema bag with lukewarm purified water and hang approximately eighteen to twenty-four inches above the floor (from towel rack or door handle).

3. Lubricate enema tip with oil.

4. Release a small amount of water to relieve any air pockets.

5. While kneeling, insert enema tip into anus, controlling the flow of water with the valve. If you feel you cannot hold the water, take deep breaths and close the valve until the feeling subsides.

6. Once the bag is empty, remove nozzle and lay down on floor in a comfortable position. Alternate positions—lie on your left side, then your back, and then your right side—to help move the water around.

7. Massage your abdomen, starting with descending colon (left side of lower abdomen). Work up to the transverse and then down the ascending colon (right side of abdomen).

8. When you have the urge to release, sit on the toilet (preferably with knees up on a stool).

9. Continue massaging the abdomen and remain on toilet until all water and waste is released.

Tips:
• Do not use hot water—this is a shock to the colon and can result in reabsorption of toxins.
• Warm water helps loosen solids.
• Cold water contracts muscle tissue and stimulates peristalsis (wavelike contractions that move food along the digestive tract). It can cause cramping if too cold.
• You can add wheatgrass juice or E$_3$Live to enema water (great for healing and detoxifying the colon walls).
• Without forcing yourself, try to retain the enema water for two to ten minutes.
• If the bag is suspended too high, excessive pressure can cause discomfort. The bag should be just high enough to allow water to barely flow. Don't worry how long the enema takes.
• Always breathe and relax. Follow enemas with wheatgrass implants (wheatgrass juice used as rectal implants).

Wheatgrass implants

These implants nourish the colon walls. By bypassing the stomach, they replenish the body with electrolytes and minerals (especially beneficial after colonics). Wheatgrass implants (also called retention enemas) are excellent for quickly restoring health to the body. They should be taken after an enema or colonic, the same way as enemas (with an enema bag) or with a bulb syringe (see below).

How to take an implant:
Lubricate an enema bag or bulb syringe (found at most pharmacies) with olive or castor oil. Kneel down, lowering your head and shoulders to the floor, gently squeezing four to six ounces of wheatgrass juice into the rectum. Relax and rest for as long as you feel comfortable; try for twenty to thirty minutes. If you need to release, do so, and then follow with another implant, holding as long as possible. The longer you retain the wheatgrass juice, the better. It might be challenging at first, but over time, you should be able to retain six ounces of wheatgrass successfully.

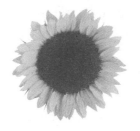

CHAPTER FOUR:
AFTER THE PROGRAM:
Maintaining a Healthy Lifestyle

COMING OFF THE PROGRAM IS AN IMPORTANT part of the detox, and it's a time to exercise diligence. Consuming large or difficult-to-digest meals will shock your system out of its cleansing mode and may cause discomfort or illness. Your digestive system will be much more sensitive than usual, and overindulging will burden your body and defeat the purpose of your cleanse.

Your taste buds will have changed during the detox, and you'll most likely crave cleaner foods, so use this opportunity to build upon the positive lifestyle habits you've cultivated over the past four weeks. Go slowly, eat small portions, and increase your food intake gradually over the upcoming days and weeks. You are now rebuilding your health.

Continue to eat high-water-content foods such as sprouts, green smoothies, juice, salads, and ripe fruit for the next three days, making sure to chew slowly and thoroughly. You may then reintroduce some heavier foods such as soaked nuts, seeds, and lightly steamed veggies. It is important to keep your meals clean and simple, staying away from complicated combinations. Remember, the more foods you eat at once, the more your digestive system has to multi-task.

Below is a sample day menu of how to maintain the lifestyle once the four-week program is completed. The raw lifestyle can vary from day to day and with the seasons. For example, one naturally craves denser, heavier foods during the winter, and intake of nuts, pâtés, milks, crackers, and avocados may increase. This allows us to add a few extra pounds of insulation against the cold temperatures.

Be sure to keep the focus on sprouts and leafy greens at all times. They are the most nourishing foods available. And remember, the foods you eliminate from your diet are as important to consider as the foods you incorporate. Meat, dairy, and all animal products are acid-forming and produce mucus in the body. They also clog up the system and can lead to various health issues. If you do eat something off the program, be sure to balance it with alkalizing, high-water-content foods.

Sample day:

Upon rising:
wheatgrass juice, E₃Live, or other concentrated green and
Lemon Water or Fire Water or
herbal tea

Breakfast:
fresh melon or other fruit or fruit smoothie or
1 quart green smoothie or green juice

Mid-morning:
2 tbsp bee pollen and
juice or smoothie with Vitamineral™ Green or
sprouted cereal

Lunch:
1 quart green smoothie or large sprout salad and
seed cheese with veggie sticks or
dehydrated crackers with hemp or flax butter

Afternoon snack:
1–2 oz wheatgrass juice or
hemp milkshake

☾ Dinner:
Energy Soup with Flax Cream or Spinach Soup and/or
Zucchini Noodles with Marinara Sauce or
large mixed green salad with sprouts and sunflower pâté or
lightly steamed veggies (optional)
Evening snack:
apple slices with 1 tbsp almond butter or dulse or
Carrot Cake with Cashew Cheese Icing (see recipe in Appendix 1) or
Live Pudding with soaked chia seeds
herbal tea

A detoxification program lasts much longer than just the duration of your cleanse. Healthy lifestyle habits need to be maintained daily in order to keep your body clean and well nourished. Now that you have rid your body of many toxins, have lost weight and feel great, you'll want to sustain this by continuing to eat fresh, ripe, whole, organic foods. After completing the SimplyRaw Detox Program, it will be easier to break unhealthy habits and patterns and replace them with new, health-promoting ones. If you like the way you look and feel, why return to an unhealthy lifestyle only to have to detoxify again?

Our bodies are constantly detoxifying, and it is important to cultivate eating habits that will help with this process daily, rather than occasional "quick-fix" diets. Support this continual detox process daily by eating health-promoting foods that also supply your body with vital nutrients. The more efficiently the body detoxifies daily, the less toxins are stored and the easier each detox program becomes. As your body becomes cleaner, your eating habits will change, and you will become more sensitive to harmful foods. Over time you will notice just how much or little high-quality food your body truly needs in order to be healthy.

Let your detox program be the beginning of a new, healthier life. Diet and lifestyle choices directly impact our health and quality of life, and the goal should be to keep the body cleansed, nourished, and free of toxic matter to ensure a healthier, longer, and more youthful life. To make a significant difference in our health, we must stop eating health-damaging processed foods.

Continue to avoid (or at least minimize) caffeine, alcohol, meat, dairy, wheat, sugar, cooked fats, and all processed foods. Be consistent with water intake, and stay away from refined carbohydrates and sugars, while, giving the body what it needs to build strong new tissues.

Our bodies can detoxify and self-heal efficiently. In our toxic environment, prevention should be the most important principle of health, and we need to be proactive to support and strengthen our immune system. We often take our well-being for granted until it's too late. Why not invest in our health and future now by making healthier choices? It may require self-discipline, but these efforts will have a positive outcome on our health, wellness, and quality of life. We are responsible for our own healthy futures.

Maintaining a healthy lifestyle

Maintaining an all-raw diet can be challenging for most people, so try to focus on a whole, vegan, healthy balance of mostly raw foods (ideally, 80 percent raw, 20 percent cooked). This will allow some social leeway to enjoy dinners out with friends and family as this tends to be the biggest challenge for many raw foodists. Dietary transition is an unfolding, evolving process, which can be a wonderful journey in many positive ways. It requires patience and listening to the body's needs. There's no need to become stressed or rigid over your eating habits. Find a healthy comfort level and make improvements slowly and consistently from there. Time will take care of the rest.

While eating completely raw might not be for everyone, maintaining a high amount of raw and living foods in our diet is beneficial for most of us, as the enzymes and nutrients are at their peak. You might revert to old ways of eating once in awhile for short periods of time (vacation, parties, stress, business meetings), but you can use the guidelines in this manual to help you sustain your health.

To ensure that you get the necessary nutrients for optimal health, continue eating lightly, especially before noon, and make sure to manage life's stresses by taking time to relax and breathe, preferably outdoors. Do not overeat. Exercise at least thirty minutes a day, five times a week.

No single food plan is right for everyone. Whatever path you take on your journey to health, one of the most important things is to experiment with what works best for you by listening to your body's signals. Take time to learn about nutrition and do the best you can, eating high-quality foods as a permanent part of your diet. Practice healthy lifestyle choices. You deserve it.

Key elements to healthy living

Incorporate the following into your lifestyle:

- Drink half your body weight in ounces of purified water each day.
- Do not drink water *with* meals, as this can dilute the digestive juices (drink one-half hour before or after eating).
- Drink one quart of fresh green smoothies daily.
- Eat only fresh foods; avoid all packaged, prepared, or fast foods.
- Eat Energy Soup daily.
- Juice sprouts and greens regularly.
- Include as many fresh green vegetables and sprouts in your daily diet as possible.
- Do not eat unripe fruit.
- Drink two to three ounces of wheatgrass juice daily.
- Have one to two tablespoons of concentrated greens daily.
- Eat two to four heaping tablespoons of live sauerkraut each day.

- Avoid refined sugars and processed starches.
- Eat small meals regularly throughout the day to maintain blood sugar levels and keep your metabolism active.
- Keep meals simple by not mixing too many foods together.
- Chew your food thoroughly, mixing well with saliva.
- Eat sea vegetables for trace elements, amino acids, minerals, and essential fatty acids.
- Have at least one tablespoon of essential fatty acids to help support your cardiovascular, immune, reproductive, and nervous systems. Good vegetarian sources of EFAs include soaked flax, chia, and hemp seeds, flax, borage, evening primrose, and hemp oils.
- Supplement your digestive system daily with plant-based digestive enzymes and probiotics.

Tips for a healthy lifestyle:

- Choose fresh organic foods.
- Eat only when hungry, and do not overeat.
- Always eat slowly and while seated, in a relaxed environment.
- Chew your food thoroughly.
- Eat consciously. This leads to good digestion and awareness.
- Do not mix too many foods at the same meal.

- Avoid eating at least two hours before going to bed.
- Vary your foods every day to provide your body with a broader array of nutrients.
- Your bowels should move at least twice daily, depending on the number of meals (ideally after every meal).
- Exercise regularly to provide strength, endurance, flexibility, relaxation, and enjoyment.

- Practice yoga, deep breathing, and/or meditation daily.
- Laugh as often as possible. It reduces stress and feels great.
- Ensure that you get good quality and duration of sleep.
- Practice systematic undereating.
- Detox with the seasons to eliminate accumulated waste and improve digestion and absorption.
- Avoid cleaning products made with synthetic chemicals.
- Keep the colon clean.
- Juice fast one day every week to give your digestive organs a rest.
- Trust your body to heal itself.

Acid-alkaline balance

Your food intake should ideally be 80 percent alkaline and 20 percent acid. The average western diet is too acidic, and some nutritionists believe an acidic diet creates imbalances, toxicity, inflammation, and congestion in the body. Foods such as meat, eggs, dairy, refined foods, white flour, sugar, coffee, and soft drinks are acid forming and can create acidosis (when blood pH falls below 7.35). Other factors contributing to high acidity include emotional stress, toxic overload, drugs, and excessive or too little exercise.

Too many acid-forming foods can destroy the body's delicate pH balance. When the body is too acidic, calcium is pulled out of the bones to maintain blood pH. The result is poor body function and deficiencies in minerals such as calcium, magnesium, potassium, and sodium. Acid-forming foods also contribute to health problems such as yeast overgrowth, depression, osteoporosis, joint pain and inflammation, premature aging, weight gain, ulcers, diabetes, heart disease, and cancer.

During the SimplyRaw Living Foods Detox Program, it is important to reduce the consumption of acid-forming foods and eat a lot of fresh whole foods that have a higher alkaline pH level. Alkaline-forming foods contain higher levels of calcium, potassium, magnesium, and sodium, and are generally found in most fresh, high-water-content fruits, vegetables, leafy greens, and soaked almonds.

Optimal pH balance is within the 7.35 to 7.45 range, and can easily be tested through the saliva or urine with litmus strips (available at most health food stores and pharmacies).

Alkaline and acid foods and activities:

HIGHLY ALKALINE	ALKALINE	ACIDIC	HIGHLY ACIDIC
wheatgrass juice	arugula	cooked vegetables	meat
sprouts	sweet potatoes	whole unrefined grains	cheese
Energy Soup	beets		pasteurized milk
kale	celery	sprouted grain breads	yogurt
cucumber	lettuce	raw milk products	processed foods
fresh green juice and smoothies	raw spinach	cooked spinach	food additives
	garlic	unripe fruit	refined sugar
fresh leafy greens	avocados	blueberries	refined wheat
parsley	tomatoes	cranberries	white rice
broccoli	melons	prunes	trans-, hydrogenated, and heated fats
asparagus	apples	pineapples	
sea vegetables	pears	pasteurized fruit juices	breads
grapefruits	grapes		breakfast cereals
lemons, limes	cherries	lentils	pasta
figs	almonds, soaked	chickpeas	soy sauce, tamari
watermelon	flax, chia seeds	sunflower seeds	white vinegar
papayas	hemp	pumpkin seeds	table salt
ginger	pine nuts	sesame seeds	condiments
stevia	millet	walnuts	chocolate
sunshine	amaranth	brazil nuts	candy
fresh clean air	buckwheat	cashews	peanuts
laughter	quinoa	brown rice	pistachios
deep breathing	wild rice	oats	soy and whey protein isolates
	apple cider vinegar	spelt	soft drinks
	herbal teas	popcorn	coffee, black tea
	fresh coconut water		nicotine
			drugs
			alcohol
			stress
			exercise

To learn more about acid-alkaline balance, read *The Acid-Alkaline Diet* by Christopher Vasey (Inner Traditions/Bear & Company, 2006).

Food combining

Good digestion is vital to good health. It isn't so much what we eat that is crucial to our health, but what we digest and assimilate. If your food doesn't break down, it will putrefy, and your body will absorb its own waste before it can be eliminated. Indigestion is an underlying cause of many health problems and can be avoided by not overloading the body with too many foods. Consuming too many incompatible foods can create symptoms such as lack of energy, bloating, flatulence, burping, body odor, candida, fatigue, acidity, or lower-back ache.

Food combining is based on the theory that different types of food require different lengths of time, different enzymes, and different pH balances for proper digestion. It is believed that the body is not designed to digest more than one concentrated food in the stomach at the same time. (Any food other than a fruit or vegetable is considered concentrated.)

The simpler the meal, the better you feel!

Good food combining places less of a burden on your digestive system, which means that ultimately, you'll have a higher energy level. You'll also have better absorption and less bloating and gas. Allow time between meals for your system to assimilate and rest. When eating a raw diet, one can be less stringent with food combining principles. For example, leafy greens can be combined with small amounts of fruit, especially when blended. Test the guidelines out and learn for yourself. (See page 108 for a food combining chart, and read *Fit for Life* by Harvey and Marilyn Diamond [Warner Books, 1987] for more information.)

Simple food combining principles:

1. Drink liquids alone or before meals; wait at least 15 minutes before eating.
2. Do not mix protein and carbohydrates at the same meal.
3. Eat one type of protein per meal.
4. Do not mix fats and proteins at the same meal. (Foods such as nuts are over 50 percent fat and require hours for digestion.)
5. Eat fruit alone on an empty stomach (either thirty minutes before a meal or two-and-a-half hours after) or blended with leafy greens. Fruit digestion is extremely quick but will be slowed down if eaten with other foods, causing fermentation.
6. Do not mix fruit with protein.
7. Do not eat acidic fruit with sweet fruit.
8. Eat melons alone.
9. Avoid overeating.

High-quality food combined well leads to good digestion and improved health.

If you experience gas, constipation, bloating, or tiredness after eating, these are signs that combinations can be improved and the amount of food decreased.

Food Combining Simplified

One food at a meal is ideal for the easiest and best digestion.
A combination of several foods at a meal should be according to the chart below.

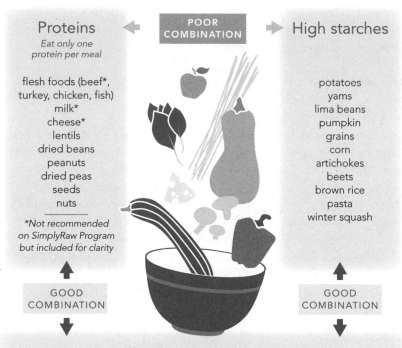

Proteins

*Eat only one
protein per meal*

POOR COMBINATION

High starches

flesh foods (beef*,
turkey, chicken, fish)
milk*
cheese*
lentils
dried beans
peanuts
dried peas
seeds
nuts

*Not recommended
on SimplyRaw Program
but included for clarity*

potatoes
yams
lima beans
pumpkin
grains
corn
artichokes
beets
brown rice
pasta
winter squash

GOOD COMBINATION

GOOD COMBINATION

Green and Low Starch Vegetables

asparagus	kohlrabi	• Tomatoes may be combined with low-starch vegetables and either nuts or avocados.
bean sprouts	mushrooms	
Brussels sprouts	okra	
broccoli	olives	• Avocados are best combined with low-starch vegetables. (They make "fair" combinations with starches.)
cabbage	peppers	
cauliflower	radishes	
celery	rhubarb	EAT ONLY FRESH FRUITS FOR BREAKFAST
cucumbers	sauerkraut	
eggplant	spinach	• Eat only one kind of fruit at a time, as much as you want.
endive	string beans	
escarole	summer squash	• Wait one hour, then eat another kind if you so desire.
leaf lettuce	swiss chard	
greens	watercress	• Stop one hour before lunch.
leeks	sea vegetables	• Melons are best eaten alone.

Quick-transit foods

The amount of time food remains in the stomach varies. Food and food combinations should have a quick transit time, otherwise the body expends energy to break these foods down and eventually stores waste from food that is not fully eliminated. This energy could otherwise be used for more supportive healing tasks within the body. On the other hand, quick-transit foods pass easily through the stomach and require less energy to digest. These foods provide us with more energy than they use.

The longer a food remains inside you, the more that food takes energy from you. If you're interested in weight loss and having more energy, follow the quick-transit principles and keep meal combinations as simple as possible.

The healthiest, most hydrating foods—fresh, raw fruits, vegetables, and juices—are also the quickest transit foods, offering the body maximum enzymes, oxygen, and chlorophyll without slowing you down.

Examples of food transit time

water	10–15 minutes
fresh juice	15–30 minutes
Rejuvelac	20–30 minutes
fresh fruit	30–60 minutes
wheatgrass juice	30–60 minutes
sprouts	1 hour
most vegetables	1–2 hours
grains, beans	1–2 hours
fatty plant foods (avocados, nuts, seeds)	2–3 hours
vegetable protein	3 hours
whole grain pastas, cereals	3–4 hours
meat, fish	3–4 hours
shellfish	8 hours

Supplementing

While we try to rely on fresh food sources to meet our daily nutritional requirements, it is often challenging to do so due to poor absorption as well as soil depletion. It has been found that using chemical fertilizers over many years can greatly reduce the nutrient level of most soils and crops. Studies show that many fruits and vegetables have lower levels of nutrients than they did fifty years ago.

Vitamins, minerals, and essential fatty acids

Vitamin B$_{12}$: Crucial for the proper functioning of the brain, the entire nervous system, and the formation of our blood, vitamin B$_{12}$, plays an important part in the metabolism of every cell in our body.

A common argument against vegetarianism is that it leads to a deficiency in vitamin B$_{12}$. However, according to many health experts, including Dr Brian Clement and Gabriel Cousens, MD, *both vegetarians and meat eaters can experience B$_{12}$ deficiency.* Vitamin B$_{12}$ is produced by bacteria in the intestines. Dr Clement recommends supplementing with a high quality, bacterial form of B$_{12}$.

In the past, some non-animal items such as spirulina, chlorella, tempeh, miso, and even soil were considered as possible sources of B$_{12}$, but these have proven to be unreliable.

Calcium: Vital for the formation of strong bones and teeth, calcium is also essential for maintenance of a regular heartbeat and muscular growth. Rich plant food sources include dark leafy greens (broccoli, bok choy, kale, collards, turnip greens, dandelion), tahini, legumes, sesame seeds, almonds, figs, seaweeds, and unrefined molasses. Since the consumption of animal protein may increase calcium requirements, a person following a vegan diet may have much lower needs.

Vitamin D: Traditionally, people have looked to fish oil for vitamin D, which is needed to maintain proper calcium levels, both in the bones and in the bloodstream. However, the best source is sunshine. Ultraviolet rays trigger vitamin D synthesis in the skin. Sun exposure of just fifteen to twenty minutes daily (early morning or late afternoon) will help provide the body with adequate stores of vitamin D. For individuals with limited sun exposure, it is important to take a good supplement.

Iodine: Needed only in trace amounts, iodine helps metabolize excess fat and is important for physical and mental health. It is vital for good thyroid function, which in turn is essential for good health. The best vegetarian sources are dulse, nori, arame, vegetables grown near the ocean, and many vitamin and mineral supplements.

Iron: A trace element needed for the formation of blood, iron is vital for the health of cells and for the transport of oxygen to all parts of the body. The richest plant sources are sea vegetables, leafy greens, beets, cherries, lentils, legumes, dried fruits, nuts (almonds, brazil nuts, cashews), seeds (pumpkin, sunflower, sesame), whole grains, and blackstrap molasses. (Adding fruits and vegetables high in vitamin C to your meals enhances iron absorption. Dairy products, on the other hand, can inhibit absorption of iron.)

Essential fatty acids: Necessary for every living cell in the body, essential fatty acids help rebuild cells. Some excellent vegetarian sources are algaes, hemp seeds and oil, flax seeds and oil, primrose and borage oils, chia seeds, and most raw nuts and seeds.

Zinc: An essential mineral required for prostate gland function, growth of reproductive organs, and protein synthesis, zinc promotes a healthy immune system and healing of wounds. Found in kelp, nuts, seeds (especially pumpkin seeds), lentils, mushrooms, and brewer's yeast.

To ensure nutritional support, complement your diet with a high quality, whole food supplement. Whole food supplements can vary in quality. The following are whole, minimally processed, and of excellent quality.

Whole food supplements

Chlorella: A single-celled freshwater grown algae, chlorella is a complete protein (approximately 58 percent), containing vitamins B, C, and E, beta-carotene, trace minerals, calcium, magnesium, zinc, potassium, and omega-3 fatty acids. It is nature's richest source of chlorophyll and commonly recommended to aid the body in the elimination of heavy metals such as mercury, cadmium, and lead. (Broken cell-wall chlorella is nearly twice as digestible as other chlorella.) Chlorella is also excellent for regulating blood sugar.

E₃Live: Minimally processed, aphanizomenon flos-aquae (AFA)—blue-green algae—this product contains high-quality amino acids, live enzymes, chlorophyll, minerals, vitamins, and essential fatty acids. E₃Live is very easily assimilated by the body. It is an excellent food to help heal and nourish your body.

Maca: Rich in calcium, magnesium, phosphorous and iron, maca increases energy and supports the immune system. It is also a hormone-balancing adaptogen that helps regulate hormones in both men and women, reduces stress, and enhances the libido.

Full spectrum plant-based enzymes: The most popular enzymes found in natural food supplements, plant-based enzymes are useful in supporting optimal digestion. They are an essential supplement when consuming heavier foods (both cooked and raw).

Probiotics: A good bacteria naturally found in the body, probiotics help support a healthy digestive system. They can be found in Rejuvelac, live sauerkraut, and other fermented foods that contain active cultures. (Look for dairy-free probiotics.)

Spirulina: A tiny aquatic plant with a remarkable concentration of nutrients including protein (65 percent), beta carotene, B-complex vitamins, vitamin E, essential trace minerals, and gamma-linolenic acid (GLA), spirulina is also a major source of iron and calcium.

Vitamineral™ Green: This product includes a full spectrum of naturally occurring, absorbable, and nontoxic vitamins, minerals (including calcium), and trace minerals. It contains no synthetic or isolated nutrients.

Schinoussa Sea Vegetables™: A raw superfood made with spirulina, chlorella, blue-green algae (E₃Live), irish moss, and dulse. This blend is clinically tested and proven to reduce free radicals within weeks if taken regularly.

Whole foods to add to your daily diet

Bee pollen: A complete food said to contain approximately 185 nutrients, including twenty-two amino acids, plus vitamins, minerals, and enzymes, it is useful for treating fatigue, hay fever, sinusitis, environmental allergies, prostate enlargement, chronic infection, and nutritional deficiencies. (People who are allergic to bees should never take bee pollen.)

Chia seeds: The richest plant source of omega-3 fatty acids, they are also an excellent source of protein, minerals, fiber, vitamin B, and antioxidants. Eat one to two tablespoons of soaked chia seeds daily.

Flax seeds: High in lignans and omega-3s, flax seeds also provide excellent nutrition in the form of protein, lecithin, minerals, vitamins, and fiber. Flax is an important food to eat daily (soak and blend). One heaping tablespoon contains two grams of alpha-linolenic acid.

Garlic: Long known for its many health benefits and medicinal properties, garlic is an antiviral, antifungal, antibacterial agent and is known to expel intestinal parasites from the body. Garlic improves circulation and lowers blood pressure and cholesterol.

Hemp seeds: As a complete protein, hemp seeds are an excellent source of amino acids and have a well-balanced ratio of omega-3 to omega-6 essential fatty acids Hemp seeds are excellent in salads and smoothies and can be made into a delicious hemp milk.

Wheatgrass juice: High in minerals, amino acids, enzymes, and vitamins A, B-complex, C, E, and K, wheatgrass juice is very helpful in strengthening the immune system. It is also a powerful blood cleanser and can help remove toxins from the blood stream.

Dulse, wakame, hijiki, and other sea vegetables: Dulse is a whole food that is high in trace elements, minerals, and iodine. It is excellent for removing toxins from the body. Be sure to soak for one minute and drain before eating. (Store in the refrigerator after soaking.) Highly alkaline sea vegetables are packed with B vitamins, minerals, iodine, and selenium to support the health and proper function of the thyroid and adrenal glands. Rich in alginates, sea vegetables are useful in removing toxins from the body. They also contain cancer-fighting lignans.

Herbal teas

While herbal teas are not considered raw foods, nor are they an essential part of the SimplyRaw Detox, I have included a variety of detox-friendly teas for those who wish to use them. Herbal teas can be very comforting and soothing to drink throughout the detox program, especially during the colder months.

Herbal teas have been used for many centuries as part of various herbal cleansing programs because of their medicinal properties. They can support the cleansing process, and some teas may help strengthen specific organs or alleviate various conditions. Herbal teas often contain high levels of antioxidants, which can be beneficial to the immune system.

When purchasing teas, choose only the highest quality organic leaves, otherwise you'll be introducing chemicals into your body.

These are some of my favorite detox teas:

Alfalfa: High in vitamins and minerals, alfalfa enhances immune function. It alkalizes, detoxifies, and purifies the bloodstream and liver, and helps fight infection.

Burdock root: One of the most popular internal cleansing herbs, burdock clears the bloodstream of toxins, stimulates the liver, regulates blood sugar, and helps eliminate uric acid from the body. It is rich in vitamins and antioxidants and is an excellent immune booster.

Cat's claw: This herb stimulates the immune system, promotes healing of wounds, and reduces inflammation and arthritis. Also helpful in treating candida, chronic fatigue, digestive troubles, bowel disorders, and viral infections.

Cayenne: The fiery red pepper known as cayenne aids digestion, improves circulation, and is very helpful for the heart, lungs, kidneys, and stomach. Add to lemon juice to make Fire Water (see recipe in Appendix 1).

Chamomile: Often used to treat digestive disorders and heartburn, chamomile is also used to alleviate stress, sleep disorders, headaches, and menstrual cramps.

Dandelion: A gentle diuretic, dandelion is also an expectorant, blood purifier, and liver cleanser. Rich in vitamins and minerals, dandelion helps with anemia, kidney function, hypoglycemia, and liver, gall bladder, and stomach problems. Dandelion leaves mixed with milk thistle make the ultimate liver detoxifier and protector.

Echinacea: Often used for fighting infections, colds, flu, sore throat, inflammation, and congestion, echinacea stimulates the white blood cells and helps speed recovery.

Fennel: Rich in phytoestrogens, fennel is commonly used for colic, indigestion, gas, asthma, congestion in the lungs, water retention, and problems in the bowels, liver, kidneys, and spleen. It is also used as an appetite suppressant and to promote milk flow in mothers.

Ginger: This spice has been traditionally used to treat indigestion, gas, stomach cramps, nausea, motion sickness, inflammation, circulation, colds, flu, and coughs.

Globe artichoke: A natural remedy for indigestion, liver, and gall bladder issues, it has also been used in traditional treatments for high cholesterol and kidney disease.

Hawthorn berry: This red berry protects against cardiovascular disease and circulatory disorders. It helps lower blood pressure and cholesterol levels. High in antioxidants, it is helpful in treating anemia.

Juniper berry: A mild diuretic, juniper berries support urinary tract health. They also aid digestion, help reduce inflammation, indigestion, and kidney and bladder issues.

Licorice root: Used to alleviate gas, heartburn, indigestion, ulcers and colic, licorice has anti-inflammatory properties and helps improve circulation. It has also been used to clear the bronchial tubes, throat, and lungs.

Milk thistle: One of the most effective herbs for relieving liver disorders, milk thistle is very high in antioxidants. It protects the liver and prevents free-radical damage. It is the ultimate liver detoxifier and protector, especially when mixed with dandelion.

Mullein: Recommended for clearing congestion, sore throats, coughs, colds, bronchitis, asthma and ear aches, mullein also acts as a laxative and sleep aid.

Nettle: This prickly herb acts as a diuretic and supports the kidneys and urinary system. It is good for clearing phlegm in the lungs and bronchial tubes. Nettle is nutritious and has been used traditionally to treat anemia.

Oregano, wild: The fragrant oil of this herb boosts the immune system and fights free radicals and infection. Oregano oil has antibacterial, antifungal, antiparasitic, and antioxidant abilities.

Parsley leaf: Its high vitamin C content makes parsley an excellent immune builder; it also improves kidney activity and helps eliminate waste from the blood. Parsley has been used to relieve gas, indigestion, bladder issues, and fluid retention.

Peppermint: Used to soothe indigestion, nausea, headaches, and poor appetite, peppermint leaves also help relieve cold or flu symptoms.

Red clover: An excellent blood purifier, red clover is also an expectorant and immune builder, and often used in treating arthritis, infections, skin diseases, toxicity, and inflammation of the urinary tract.

Rose hips: An excellent source of rutin and vitamins C, E, and A, rose hip tea helps treat and prevent bladder infections.

Taheebo: With antifungal and antibacterial properties, taheebo (also known as pau d'arco) is often used to treat candida, intestinal problems, skin issues, herpes, and viral and fungal infections. It is an excellent tea for the immune system.

Thyme, wild: Often used as a culinary herb, wild thyme is also a natural antiseptic for sore throats and coughs.

Turmeric: Useful in the treatment of arthritis, turmeric also protects the liver, helps circulation, and fights free radicals.

Valerian: Well-known for its sedative qualities, valerian is very helpful in promoting calmness and sleep without adverse side effects.

Vervain: Effective in treating migraines and headaches, vervain also acts as a mild sedative and helps cleanse the liver and gall bladder.

Yarrow: A remedy for indigestion, gas, heartburn, and stomach cramps, yarrow is also helpful for urinary infections, and gall bladder and liver conditions.

Yellow dock: Very high in iron, yellow dock acts as a blood purifier and cleanser and is an excellent remedy for treating anemia. Also supports liver and colon function.

APPENDICES

"To eat is a necessity, but to eat intelligently is an art."
—La Rochefoucauld

Recipes

The following raw recipes are simple to prepare and will help you get started on the SimplyRaw Living Foods Detox Program. Make sure to try out new recipes on a regular basis to keep yourself interested and nourished. Variety is the key!

Fresh juices and fruit smoothies
Green smoothies
Nut and seed milks
Puddings and live puddings
Breakfasts
Soups
Salads, salad dressings, and no-oil salad dressings
Pâtés, dips, and spreads
Entrees
Desserts

Fresh Juices and Fruit Smoothies

Note: If a recipe calls for lemon or lime juice, it should be fresh, not bottled; if fruit is recommended, it should be ripe and fresh unless otherwise indicated. All products should be organic, if possible.

FIRE WATER

This morning drink helps with elimination and is an excellent liver tonic. It is a great way to start the day.

• 10 oz purified water (hot or cold)
• ½ lemon, juiced
• sprinkle of cayenne

Squeeze lemon into a glass. Add water and a sprinkle of cayenne powder.

Makes 1 serving.

LEMON WATER

This drink is great for helping to kick a caffeine habit.

• juice of 1 lemon or lime
• 1 tbsp honey, raw agave, or a drop of stevia (optional)
• 2 cups water
• 1 crushed mint leaf (optional)

Mix all ingredients together and drink throughout the day.

Makes 1 serving.

CITRUS DRINK

• 2 oranges, peeled and seeded
• 1 tbsp raw agave
• 1 cup grain Rejuvelac or purified water
• 1 small avocado, peeled (optional—provides creamier texture)

Blend all ingredients.

Makes 1 serving.

GREEN JUICE

• 2 cucumbers
• 6 stalks celery
• two large handfuls of any sprouts (sunflower, alfalfa and/or pea)
• 4 kale leaves (optional)

Juice all ingredients in a juicer.

Makes 1 serving.

DR ANN'S "WAKE-UP" MORNING DRINK

Refreshing and an excellent tonic for the kidneys

• 4 cups watermelon strips (rind can be left on if organic)

Process watermelon in a juicer. Pour into tall glasses and enjoy.

Makes 1 serving.

PINEAPPLE-BANANA DRINK

• 2 cups pineapple, chopped
• ½ cup grain Rejuvelac or purified water
• 1 banana, peeled
• 1 avocado, peeled (optional—makes a creamier texture)

Blend all ingredients.

Makes 1 serving.

ORANGE GREEN

- 6 kale leaves
- 1 cup fresh orange juice
- 1 dash cayenne pepper

Blend all ingredients until creamy.

Makes 1 serving.

DR ANN'S WATERMELON SMOOTHIE

- 2 cups chopped watermelon, rind and seeds removed
- ½ cup Rejuvelac or purified water
- 1 small avocado, peeled and chopped

Blend watermelon with Rejuvelac gradually. Add avocado.

Makes 1 serving.

CARROT-APPLE SHAKE

- 1 cup fresh carrot juice
- 1 cup fresh apple juice
- 1 avocado, peeled
- squeeze of lemon

Blend ingredients together.

Makes 1 serving.

BANANA SHAKE

- 2 fresh bananas, peeled
- 2 frozen bananas, peeled
- 2 cups pure water

Blend all ingredients together.

Makes 2 servings.

CAROB SHAKE

- 2 bananas, peeled
- 2 cups purified water (cold)
- 2 tsp raw carob powder
- 1 tsp raw agave or a drop of stevia (optional)

Blend all ingredients together.

Makes 1 serving.

BERRY SMOOTHIE

- 2 cup purified water
- 1 cup fresh or frozen strawberries or blueberries
- 1 banana, peeled
- 1 tsp raw agave (optional)

Blend all ingredients on medium speed until smooth. Serve immediately.

Makes 1 serving.

Green Smoothies

Fresh green smoothies are an excellent way of adding large quantities of raw greens to your diet. They are the key to achieving optimal health and ensure that you receive high-quality nutrition in an easy-to-digest form. Made mainly from fresh leafy greens, sprouts, and fruit, they are rich in enzymes, minerals, chlorophyll, and phytonutrients that assist the body in detoxification and healing.

Use the recipes following only as guidelines. You may add concentrated greens and other superfoods to your smoothies for extra nutrition. Ease into the greens and sprouts as the taste can be overwhelmingly "earthy" and put you off smoothies in general. For beginners, start with a ratio of 60 percent fruit to 40 percent leafy greens and increase to a ratio of at least 60 percent greens to 40 percent fruit, with water to thin it down. I add only one or two pieces of fruit to my smoothies just to help remove the bitterness of some greens.

Favorite extras that I add to my smoothies include: hemp seeds, soaked flax seeds, Flax Cream, soaked chia seeds, raw maca, Vitamineral™ Green, bee pollen, flax or hemp oil, MSM powder[1], or soaked goji berries. Smoothies vary each day depending on what greens are in season and in the fridge. My green smoothies don't feel complete without sprouts.

---

1. Methylsulfonylmethane (MSM) powder has been used as an anti-inflammatory dietary supplement helpful in relieving symptoms of osteoarthritis.

MANGO-SPINACH

• 2 large mangoes, peeled and seeded
• 2 cups spinach
• water, to thin

Blend all ingredients together.

Makes 1 serving.

MELLOW GREEN SMOOTHIE

• 2 cups water
• 2 bananas, peeled
• 2 pears, cored
• 2 cups of spinach

Blend all ingredients well and enjoy!

Makes 1 serving.

RAW FAMILY WILD BANANGO

• 2 cups lambsquarter (or substitute plantain or chickweed)
• 1 banana, peeled
• 1 mango, peeled and seeded
• 2 cups water

Blend well.

Makes 1 serving.

APPLE-KALE

• 4 apples, cored
• ½ cup lemon juice
• 4 leaves kale
• water to thin

Blend all ingredients together.

Makes 1 serving.

MINTY KALE AND PEAR

- 4 ripe pears
- 5 leaves kale
- ½ bunch mint
- water to thin

Blend all ingredients together.

Makes 1 serving.

ORANGE BANANA

- 1 cup freshly squeezed orange juice
- 2 bananas, peeled
- ½ bunch romaine lettuce

Blend all ingredients together.

Makes 1 serving.

NATASHA'S MID-MORNING REFRESHER

- 1 cup freshly pressed pineapple juice
- ½-inch piece ginger, ½-inch thick
- 1 cup water
- 1 heaping tbsp Vitamineral™ Green
- 1 banana, peeled

Process pineapple and ginger in juicer. Then add all ingredients to blender, blending until smooth.

Makes 1 serving.

GREEN POWER

- 1 cup water
- 2 stalks celery
- ½ small cucumber
- 1-inch piece ginger, 1-inch thick
- 2 cups spinach
- ½ small pineapple, peeled and cored
- ½ lemon, peeled
- small handful of ice

Blend all ingredients until smooth.

Makes 1 large serving.

POWER MORNING SHAKE

Just one-quarter cup of walnuts provides you with a day's worth of omega-3 fatty acids. If you're allergic to nuts, use a tablespoon of ground flax or hemp seeds instead.

- 1 banana, frozen or fresh, peeled
- 1 cup berries, frozen or fresh
- ¼ cup walnuts, soaked overnight
- 1 tbsp green powder

Blend until smooth.

Makes 1 serving.

NATASHA'S VERY GREEN SUPER SMOOTHIE

This will keep you going for hours. Pour into thermos and bring along with you.

- 2 cups purified water
- 1 banana, peeled (optional)
- ½–1 whole head romaine lettuce
- ½ cucumber, chopped
- handful sunflower sprouts (greens)
- handful cilantro
- 1 tbsp raw maca
- 2 tbsp soaked chia seeds
- 1 tbsp Vitamineral™ Green
- 1 tbsp bee pollen
- 1 tsp MSM powder

Blend all ingredients until smooth. Thin with water if necessary.

Makes 1 serving.

SIMPLYRAW'S SPRING SMOOTHIE

May is for mango … smoothies!

- 2 mangoes, peeled and seeded
- 2 cups water
- 1 head spinach
- large handful sunflower sprouts (greens)
- 2–3 dandelion leaves (optional)

Blend all ingredients.

Makes 1 serving.

SIMPLYRAW'S SUN-FILLED SMOOTHIE

- 1 cup freshly pressed orange juice
- 1 cup purified water
- ½ banana, peeled
- 2 cups sunflower sprouts (greens)
- handful alfalfa sprouts
- 2 cups baby greens
- handful parsley leaves
- 2 tbsp soaked flax or chia seeds

Blend all ingredients until smooth.

Makes 1 serving.

SMOOTHIE ON-THE-RUN

- 2 cups purified water
- 2 ripe bananas, peeled
- handful mixed organic greens
- 1 tbsp Vitamineral™ Green
- 1 tbsp hemp seeds
- 1 tbsp raw maca

Blend all ingredients until creamy.

Makes 1 serving.

TOMATO-SPROUT ENERGY SMOOTHIE

- 3 cups ripe tomatoes, chopped
- 2 cups mixed sprouts (alfalfa, sunflower, buckwheat)
- small handful cilantro or basil
- ½ cup celery, chopped
- Himalayan salt or dulse to taste

Blend all ingredients until smooth.

Makes 2 servings.

Nut and Seed Milks

Fresh nut and seed milks are very nutritious and curb those cravings.

VANILLA ALMOND MILK

- 1 cup almonds (soaked overnight)
- 3–4 cups purified water
- 6 dates, pitted (soaked 4 hours)
- 1 tsp vanilla extract

Blend all ingredients at high speed until creamy. Strain using a nut milk bag or fine sieve. Serve over sprouted cereal, gRAWnola (see recipe, page 133), in smoothies, or alone. For a delicious eggnog alternative, simply add nutmeg, ground cloves, a banana, and pinch of salt!

Makes 4 servings.

HEMP MILK

- ¼ cup hemp seed
- 2 cups water
- ½ cup frozen berries
- 1 banana, peeled
- 1 tsp agave or a drop of stevia (to taste)

Blend all ingredients until creamy.

Makes 2 servings.

CAROB-DATE SHAKE

- 2 fresh or frozen bananas, peeled
- ¼ cup sunflower seeds, soaked overnight
- 1 cup purified water
- 2 dates, pitted (or 1 tsp agave or drop of stevia)
- 1 tbsp raw carob powder

Blend all ingredients until creamy.

Makes 2 servings.

STRAWBERRY SHAKE

- 1 tbsp raw tahini
- 1 banana, peeled (fresh or frozen)
- ½ cup strawberries (fresh or frozen)
- 2 cups almond milk
- 1 tbsp concentrated greens (E₃Live, barley grass, blue-green algae, spirulina, chlorella)

Blend all ingredients together.

Makes 2 servings.

BLUEBERRY MILKSHAKE

- 2 cups purified water
- 2 bananas, peeled (fresh or frozen)
- ½ cup fresh or frozen blueberries
- 3 dates, pitted
- ¼ cup hemp or sunflower seeds (soaked)
- ½ tsp cinnamon
- sprinkle nutmeg

Blend all ingredients until smooth.

Makes 2 servings.

CAROB SUPER-SHAKE

- 3 cups almond milk
- 1 banana, peeled
- 3 tbsp raw carob powder
- 1 tbsp maca
- 1 tsp cinnamon
- pinch of Celtic or Himalayan salt

Process all ingredients until smooth.

Makes 2 servings.

Puddings

Fruit puddings are light, cleansing, and ideal for mornings.

MELLOW MELON PUDDING

- 2 cups cantaloupe, peeled, seeded, and chopped
- 1 cup honeydew, peeled, seeded, and chopped
- juice of 1 lime

Blend in food processor or blender until smooth.

Makes 1 serving.

BANANA-AVOCADO PUDDING

- 2 bananas, peeled
- ½ avocado, peeled and seeded

Blend until smooth.

Makes 1 serving.

PEACHY MANGO PUDDING

- 6 peaches, seeded and chopped
- 2 mangos, peeled, seeded, and chopped

Blend until smooth.

Makes 2 servings.

PERSIMMON PUDDING

- 1 ripe persimmon, seeded and chopped
- ½ cup water

Blend until smooth.

Makes 1 serving.

MANGOCADO

- 1 mango, peeled, seeded, and chopped
- ½ avocado, peeled, seeded, and chopped

Blend until smooth.

Makes 1 serving.

PAPAYA PUDDING

- 1 ripe papaya, peeled, seeded, and chopped
- 2 bananas, peeled

Blend until smooth.

Makes 1 serving.

SUMMER PUDDING

- 2 bananas, peeled
- 2 mangos
- 1 cup strawberries
- 4 dates

Process in food processor until smooth.

Makes 2 servings.

PRUNELLA

- 1 banana, peeled
- 8 prunes, soaked overnight

Process in food processor until smooth.

Makes 1 serving.

CREAMY PEAR

- 1 pear, cored and quartered
- ¼ avocado, peeled and seeded

Blend until smooth.

Makes 1 serving.

QUICK AND EASY APPLE SAUCE

- 4 apples, peeled, cored, and chopped
- 6 large dates, pitted
- ⅛ tsp cinnamon

Blend all ingredients together in food processor or blender.

Makes 2 servings.

BANANA PUDDING

- 3 ripe bananas, peeled
- ½ cup raisins, soaked 2 hours
- ¼ tsp cinnamon

Blend well in food processor or blender.

Makes 2 servings.

MANGO BERRY PARFAIT

- 2 cups mango, peeled, seeded, and chopped
- 2 tbsp coconut oil
- 1 tsp vanilla extract (or ½ vanilla bean, ground)
- 2 tbsp lime juice
- 1 tsp lime zest
- ¼ cup raw agave
- 1 cup fresh berries
- sprig of fresh mint

Blend everything except for berries and mint. Refrigerate at least 2 hours. Layer in cups with fresh berries and garnish with sprig of mint.

Makes 2 servings.

BLUE BLISS

- 2 bananas, peeled
- 1 cup blueberries
- 1 cup cherries, pitted
- ¼ cup dates, pitted

Blend all ingredients until smooth.

Makes 2 servings.

VANILLA-COCONUT CREAM

- 2 coconuts, hulled and chopped, and coconut water
- 1 whole vanilla bean (or 1 tsp vanilla extract)

Blend all ingredients well in food processor until smooth.

Makes 2 servings.

FLAX (OR CHIA) CREAM

An excellent source of omega-3s and healthy fats. Add a few spoonfuls to your bowl of Energy Soup for variety. (Do not add avocado to Energy Soup if using Flax Cream.)

- 1 part soaked golden flax (or chia) seeds
- 6 parts purified water

Blend until smooth, adding more water if necessary.

Makes 6 servings.

Living Puddings

Adding sprouts or a handful of leafy greens to puddings are an excellent way of balancing the fruit sugars with alkaline minerals.

LIVING APPLE SAUCE

- 3 apples, cored and quartered
- 2 handfuls sunflower greens

Blend apples until smooth. Add sprouts and blend again.

Makes 2 servings.

LIVE PAPAYA PUDDING

- 2 cups papaya, peeled, seeded, and chopped
- 1 cup sunflower sprouts

Blend papaya until smooth. Add sprouts and blend again.

Makes 2 servings.

BANANA-MANGO-SPINACH PUDDING

- 4 bananas, peeled
- 1–2 mangos
- 1 cup spinach (or more, to taste)

Blend until smooth.

Makes 2-4 servings.

LIVING BANANA PUDDING

- 2 bananas, peeled
- ½ avocado, peeled and seeded
- 1 cup sunflower sprouts

Blend banana and avocado until smooth. Add sprouts and blend again.

Makes 2 servings.

GREEN BANANA PUDDING

- 1 frozen banana, peeled
- 1 fresh banana, peeled
- 1 tsp Vitamineral™ Greens or spirulina
- 1 tbsp soaked chia seeds
- 1 tbsp agave
- 1 tsp vanilla extract (or sprinkle of cinnamon)
- handful goji berries (topping)
- 1 tbsp bee pollen (topping)

In food processor, combine all ingredients, reserving goji and bee pollen for topping.

Makes 2 servings.

Breakfasts

For best digestion, save the heavier breakfasts for later in the morning.

FRESH MELON SALAD

- 1 cup cantaloupe, peeled, seeded, and chopped
- 1 cup honeydew melon, peeled, seeded, and chopped
- 1 cup seedless watermelon, peeled, seeded, and chopped

Mix all ingredients and enjoy.

Makes 2 serving.

BUCKWHEAT PORRIDGE

- 1 cup sprouted buckwheat (soaked overnight and rinsed well)
- 6 dates, pitted
- 1 apple, cored and chopped
- 1 banana, peeled and chopped
- 1 tsp cinnamon
- dash nutmeg (to taste)

Mix all ingredients together.

Makes 2 servings.

LIVE OATS

A quick but hearty (late morning) breakfast.

- 1 cup raw oat groats, soaked 18 hours
- 1 cup almond milk
- 1 banana, peeled and sliced finely
- sprinkle of raw agave or maple syrup
- sprinkle of cinnamon

Rinse soaked oat groats well and mix with other ingredients.

Makes 2 servings.

CRÈME BUCKWHEAT

- 1 cup sprouted buckwheat
- ½ cup purified water
- 1 banana, peeled
- ¼ cup soaked raisins
- pinch of cinnamon

Blend buckwheat, water, and banana together. Add soaked raisins and serve. This will last up to 1 day in the fridge.

Makes 1–2 servings.

LIVING MUESLI

This will keep you energized for hours!

- 1 banana, peeled and sliced finely
- 1 tbsp soaked chopped almonds
- 1 tbsp soaked sunflower seeds
- 1 tbsp soaked pumpkin seeds
- 1 tbsp soaked chia seeds
- 1 tbsp hemp seeds
- 1 tbsp soaked raisins
- sprinkle cinnamon
- almond milk, to taste

Mix ingredients in a bowl and serve immediately.

Makes 1 serving.

SIMPLYRAW'S GRAWNOLA

A high-energy meal, best eaten (in small amounts) towards midday.

- 1 cup almonds (soaked overnight)
- 1 cup pumpkin seeds (soaked overnight)
- 1 cup sunflower seeds (soaked overnight)
- 4 tbsp flax seeds (soaked overnight)
- 4 tbsp chia seeds (soaked overnight)
- 1 cup dates, pitted and chopped (soaked 2–4 hours)
- ½ cup raisins (soaked 2–4 hours)
- 2 apples, grated
- 2 tsp cinnamon

Put everything in food processor and pulse until coarsely ground. Add raisin soak water if needed to achieve thinner consistency. Top with sliced bananas and vanilla almond milk. This can also be dehydrated and made into crunchy gRAWnola.

Makes 8 servings.

Soups

Soups are an easy way to eat more vegetables, since blending concentrates a large amount of vegetables into a small volume of soup. Blending also helps break down the fibers in vegetables, making them easier to digest—important if you are new to raw.

CREAM OF ZUCCHINI SOUP

- ½ cup water
- 1 zucchini, chopped (about 1 cup)
- 1 stalk celery, chopped
- 1 tbsp lemon juice
- 1 clove garlic
- ¼ tsp Himalayan salt or dulse
- 1 tbsp olive oil
- ½ avocado, peeled, seeded, and chopped
- 1 tsp dried dill

Place all ingredients, except olive oil, avocado, and dill, in a blender. Blend until smooth. Add olive oil and avocado, blending until creamy. Add dill and blend briefly just to mix. Serve immediately.

Makes 2 servings.

CREAMY CELERY SOUP

- 2 cups almond milk
- 2 cups celery juice
- 1 clove garlic, crushed
- 1 green onion, chopped
- ¼ cup lemon juice
- ½ tsp Himalayan salt (or dulse)

Blend all ingredients together until smooth.

Makes 2 servings.

TOMATO-CELERY SOUP

Quick, simple, and surprisingly good!

- 4 med. tomatoes, chopped
- 8 stalks celery, chopped
- 1 tbsp lime juice

Blend lightly, leaving soup chunky.

Makes 2 servings.

GAZPACHO

- 3 med. tomatoes
- 1 med. red bell pepper, seeded and diced
- 1 tbsp olive oil
- water as needed
- 1 med. cucumber, diced
- ½ cup mixed sprouts (sunflower and/or alfalfa)
- 1 tbsp herbs (basil, oregano)
- juice of 1 lemon
- Himalayan salt or dulse (to taste)

Blend tomato, pepper, oil, and water until smooth. Add cucumber, mixed sprouts and herbs. Stir in lemon juice. Season to taste.

Makes 2 servings.

CREAM OF TOMATO SOUP

- 4 Roma or 2 vine-ripened tomatoes, peeled, seeded, and chopped (about 1½ cups)
- ¼ cup water
- 1 clove garlic, crushed
- ¼ tsp Himalayan salt or dulse
- ¼ tsp onion powder
- ½ avocado, chopped
- 1 tsp dried basil

Place all ingredients except avocado and basil in a blender. Blend until smooth. Add avocado and blend until creamy. Add basil and blend briefly just to mix.

Makes 2 servings.

ANN WIGMORE'S ENERGY SOUP

This recipe can be varied by choosing from a wide selection of greens and sprouts.

- 1 cup Rejuvelac or purified water
- 1 tbsp dulse
- 1 apple, cored and chopped (optional)
- small piece of yam, chopped
- 1 cup green leafy vegetables (kale, spinach, lambsquarter leaves, collards, cilantro)
- ¼ cup sprouted legumes (lentils, peas, or mung)
- ½ cup alfalfa sprouts (or other sprouts)
- 2 cups sunflower greens (sprouts)
- ½ cup buckwheat greens (sprouts)
- ½ avocado, peeled and seeded

Blend dulse with Rejuvelac or water. Add apple and harder vegetables first, followed by greens and sprouts, saving avocado for last. Pour into bowls, and serve with chopped or blended papaya.

Makes 2–4 servings.

SPINACH-APPLE SOUP

- 1 cup water
- 1 cup apple, cored, peeled and chopped
- 4 cups spinach
- 2 tbsp lemon juice
- 1 avocado, peeled and seeded
- pinch of Himalayan salt
- sprinkle of cayenne

Blend apple and water. Add spinach and blend. Add rest of ingredients and blend again until smooth.

Makes 2 servings.

QUICK AND EASY SPINACH SOUP

- ½ cup water
- 2 cups spinach
- 1 tbsp raw tahini
- 2 tbsp sun-dried tomatoes (soaked in water at least 30 minutes)
- 1 clove garlic, crushed
- 1 tbsp onion, minced
- 1 avocado, peeled and seeded
- 2 tbsp fresh basil

Blend all ingredients until smooth.

Makes 2 servings.

CREAMY KALE SOUP

- 1 cup water
- 10 cups kale, chopped
- 2 cucumbers, chopped (if organic, don't peel)
- 1 red pepper, seeded and chopped
- juice of ½ lemon
- small handful cilantro
- 1 tbsp light unpasteurized miso
- 1 tbsp raw tahini
- 1 avocado, peeled and seeded

Place water in blender and blend with kale, cup by cup. Add remaining ingredients, continuing to blend, leaving avocado for last.

Makes 4 servings.

COOL CUCUMBER SOUP

- 2 cucumbers, peeled and chopped
- 2 stalks celery, chopped
- 1 clove garlic, crushed
- 2 tbsp lemon juice
- 1 cup sunflower sprouts
- 2 tbsp fresh cilantro
- ½ avocado, peeled and seeded
- dulse or Himalayan salt, to taste

Reserve two handfuls of chopped cucumber. Place remaining cucumber and rest of ingredients into blender, blending well. Pour into bowls and add reserved cucumber for texture.

Makes 2 servings.

CREAMY CAULIFLOWER SOUP

A heartier soup for those cold winter nights.

- 2 cups almond milk
- 1 medium cauliflower, chopped
- 1 red pepper, seeded and chopped
- ½ avocado, peeled and seeded
- juice of 1 lemon
- 2 tbsp raw tahini
- 2 tbsp unpasteurized miso
- ½ jalapeno pepper, seeded and diced
- 2 cloves garlic

Blend all ingredients until creamy.

Makes 4 servings.

SIMPLYRAW'S SPINACH DILL SOUP

This alkaline soup is delicious with flax crackers.

- 2½ cups purified water
- 2 cups peeled and chopped zucchini
- 3 cups spinach
- ½ cup cored, peeled, and chopped apple
- ½ cup chopped green onion
- 1 clove garlic, crushed
- 1 tsp unpasteurized light, mellow miso
- 1 tsp Himalayan salt (optional)
- 2 tbsp fresh lemon juice
- 1½ tbsp minced fresh dill
- ⅛ tsp black pepper
- ½ fresh avocado, peeled and seeded

Combine water, zucchini, spinach, apple, green onion, garlic, miso, salt, lemon juice, dill, and pepper and blend until smooth. Do not overblend. Add avocado and blend again until smooth (about 30 seconds).

Makes 4 servings.

INDIAN CARROT SOUP

Easy and full of flavor!

- 2 cups fresh carrot juice
- 1 ripe avocado, peeled and seeded
- 1 tbsp curry powder
- 1 clove garlic, crushed
- 1 tbsp grated ginger
- 2 tbsp chopped cilantro

Blend all ingredients except for cilantro. Garnish with cilantro.

Makes 2 servings.

MINTY PINEAPPLE SOUP

- 1 pineapple, peeled, cored, and chopped
- 1 cucumber, peeled and chopped
- 3 sprigs mint

Blend all ingredients together.

Makes 2–4 servings.

BLENDED SALAD

- 4 romaine lettuce leaves
- ½ small carrot, chopped
- ½ cucumber, chopped (if organic, don't peel)
- 1 stalk celery, chopped
- ¼ red pepper, seeded and chopped
- juice of 1 lime
- 1 clove garlic, crushed
- ½ avocado, peeled and seeded
- water to thin

Blend all ingredients until smooth.

Makes 1 serving.

Salads and Salad Dressings

Fresh salads offer vital nutrients, tastes, colors, and textures. Whether you get creative with tasty salad dressings or keep it simple with fresh lemon juice and herbs, the possibilities are endless!

SWEET BABY SPINACH SALAD

This salad goes well with Orange-Avocado Dressing.

- 1 cup chopped pineapple
- 1 orange, peeled, chopped, and seeded
- 6 handfuls baby spinach
- 1 handful sunflower greens

Place all ingredients in large bowl and toss well.

Makes 2 servings.

MIXED GREENS WITH GINGER DRESSING

- 2 cups baby greens
- 2 tomatoes, chopped
- ½ cup sprouted mung beans
- 1 cup sunflower sprouts (greens)

Dressing:
- ½ cup flax oil
- 2 tbsp raw agave
- 4 tbsp lemon juice
- 1 tbsp Nama Shoyu (optional)
- 1 tsp onion powder
- ¼-inch piece ginger, ¼-inch thick, chopped
- dash of cayenne

Blend dressing ingredients, then toss desired amount with greens. Dressing (makes about ¾ cup) will keep one week in fridge.

Makes 2 servings.

SPROUT SALAD

A power-packed salad available year round.

- 3 cups sunflower sprouts
- 1 cup alfalfa sprouts
- 1 carrot, grated
- ½ zucchini, grated
- ½ red pepper, seeded and diced
- 1 celery stalk, thinly sliced

Dressing:
- 1 tomato, chopped
- ¼ cup olive oil
- 2 tsp lemon juice
- 1 clove garlic, crushed
- ½ tsp Himalayan salt or dulse

Blend dressing ingredients and toss with salad.

Makes 2 servings.

GARDEN SALAD

- ¼ head red leaf lettuce, torn
- ¼ head Romaine lettuce, torn
- ⅛ med. cucumber, thinly sliced
- ¼ med. carrot, thinly sliced
- ¼ med. zucchini, thinly sliced
- ¼ avocado, thinly sliced
- ½ Roma tomato, in wedges
- 2 tsp lemon juice
- 2 tbsp extra-virgin olive oil

Toss all ingredients with dressing of your choice. Serve immediately.

Makes 2–4 servings.

KALE SALAD

Very quick, nutritious, and delicious!

- 1 head kale, shredded
- 1 cup chopped tomato
- 1 avocado, peeled, seeded, and cubed

Dressing:
- 2 tbsp olive oil (optional)
- 1 tbsp lemon juice
- Himalayan salt, to taste (optional)
- dash of cayenne

Mix dressing ingredients, toss well with salad, and marinate 1 hour or until tender.

Makes 2 servings.

SPICY KALE SALAD

- 1 bunch organic kale, finely chopped
- 2 tbsp goji berries
- 1 cup mung or lentil sprouts
- 2 green onions, sliced finely

Dressing:
- 2 tbsp lemon juice
- 2 tbsp flax or hemp oil
- Himalayan salt to taste (optional)
- fresh chili pepper (to taste)
- 2 cloves garlic, minced

Blend dressing, then add to salad ingredients. Marinate for about 3 hours.

Makes 2–4 servings.

MIXED GREEN SALAD DELUXE

This is an excellent way of eating your greens.

- 1 tsp Himalayan salt
- 1 head mixed greens (collard, swiss chard, kale, stems removed and sliced very finely)
- 2 carrots, grated
- 10 cherry tomatoes, halved
- 1 avocado, peeled, seeded, and diced

Dressing:
- 3 tbsp olive oil (optional)
- 2 tbsp lemon juice
- pinch of cayenne

In large bowl, sprinkle salt on kale and massage with hands until tender. Combine with remaining ingredients and dressing. Marinate for 1 hour.

Makes 2–4 servings.

WALDORF SALAD

- 2 apples, cored and chopped
- 2 celery stalks, chopped
- handful raisins
- handful walnuts
- 2 cups romaine lettuce, torn into bite-sized pieces

Mix all ingredients (except for lettuce) together and serve on romaine leaves, tossed with dressing of your choice from the selection below.

Makes 2 servings.

EASY SPINACH SALAD

- 2 cups baby leaf spinach
- ½ cup chopped cauliflower
- ¼ cup grated carrots
- 2 tbsp sunflower seeds, soaked

Dressing:
- 2 tbsp olive oil
- 1 tsp lemon juice
- dash Celtic sea salt
- 1 clove garlic, crushed

Mix salad ingredients in a bowl and toss with dressing.

Makes 2 servings.

WIGMORE'S HEALTH SALAD

This salad is easy to prepare and packed full of enzymes.

- 1 cup sunflower or buckwheat greens
- 1 cup alfalfa or fenugreek sprouts
- ¼ cup grated zucchini
- ½ cup seeded and chopped red pepper

Mix together the greens and sprouts, arranging the vegetables on top. Top with any no-oil dressing (pages 146–147).

Makes 1 serving.

SPROUTED QUINOA SALAD

- 1 cup dry quinoa, soaked 6 hours, then sprouted 2–3 days
- 2 cups diced cucumbers
- 2 cups diced tomatoes
- 3 peeled, seeded and diced avocados

Dressing:
- juice of 1 lemon
- 2 tbsp Nama Shoyu
- 2 tbsp minced parsley

In large bowl, combine salad ingredients, add dressing, and mix well.

Makes 2 servings.

CABBAGE SLAW

- ½ red cabbage, sliced finely
- 2 med. carrots, grated
- 4 stalks celery, finely chopped

Dressing:
- 2 tbsp lime juice
- 2 tbsp raw apple cider vinegar
- 4 tbsp olive, flax, or hemp oil
- dash of cayenne
- Himalayan salt, to taste

Combine salad ingredients with dressing in large bowl. Toss well and let sit for several hours, allowing flavors to meld.

Makes 2 servings.

GRATED RED CABBAGE

- ½ head of red cabbage, grated

Dressing:
- 2 tbsp cold-pressed olive oil
- 2 tbsp lemon juice or raw cider vinegar
- ½ tsp Himalayan salt or dulse
- ¼ tsp dried basil

Combine cabbage with dressing. Adjust seasoning to taste.

Makes 2 servings.

DAIKON SALAD

Daikon is a large, white mild-flavored radish.

- 1 cup grated daikon
- ½ tsp grated ginger
- 1 tsp minced parsley

Place daikon in small serving bowl. Sprinkle with ginger and parsley.

Makes 2 servings.

Salad Dressings

CREAMY ITALIAN DRESSING

- ¾ cup olive oil
- ¼ cup raw apple cider vinegar
- 2 cloves garlic
- 2 tbsp fresh lemon juice
- 1 tsp Himalayan salt
- ½ cup fresh basil
- 1 tsp dried oregano
- ⅓ cup water

Blend all ingredients together and use for mixed salads.

Yields 2 cups.

CREAMY TAHINI DRESSING

- 4 tbsp raw tahini
- 4 tbsp warm water
- juice of 1 lemon
- 1 tbsp Nama Shoyu
- dash of cayenne

Add water to tahini and mix well with spoon. Add rest of ingredients and adjust amount of water if too thick. This dressing will thicken in the fridge.

Yields approximately ½ cup.

CREAMY TAHINI DIP

Use the same ingredients as above dressing, but with less water. Serve cauliflower, broccoli, and baby carrots with this tasty dip.

No-oil Salad Dressings

DR ANN'S DRESSING

- 2 tbsp lemon juice
- ½ ripe avocado, peeled and seeded
- ½ tsp fresh dill (optional)

Blend all together. Add more lemon for lighter taste.

Yields approximately ½ cup.

ORANGE AVOCADO DRESSING

- 1 avocado, peeled and seeded
- juice of 1 orange
- ½ tsp Nama Shoyu or tamari sauce

Blend all ingredients until smooth.

Yields approximately ½ cup.

GREEN GODDESS DRESSING

- 1 avocado, peeled and seeded
- 1 clove garlic, crushed
- juice of 1 lime
- 1 stalk celery, chopped
- 1 green onion, chopped
- ½ tsp dulse
- 2 tbsp water

Blend all ingredients until smooth. If dressing is too thick, add more water.

Yields approximately ½ cup.

VEGETABLE DRESSING

- 1 tomato, chopped
- 1 cucumber, chopped

- 1 red pepper. seeded and chopped
- 2 tbsp cilantro (or to taste)
- ½ tsp dulse
- 2 tbsp Rejuvelac or water

Blend all ingredients until smooth. If dressing is too thick, add more water or Rejuvelac. Yields 1 cup.

SWEET AND SPICY DRESSING

- ½ avocado
- 4 tbsp lemon juice
- 1 tbsp raisins (soaked at least 30 minutes)
- dash of cayenne
- Rejuvelac or water

Blend all ingredients until smooth. If dressing is too thick, add more water or Rejuvelac. Yields ½ cup.

PAPAYA DRESSING

- ½ ripe papaya, peeled and chopped
- juice of ½ lime
- dash of Himalayan salt
- 2 tbsp water

Blend all ingredients until smooth.
Yields 1 cup.

CREAMY PINEAPPLE DRESSING

- 1½ cups peeled and chopped pineapple
- ½ cup orange juice

Blend all ingredients until smooth.
Yields 2 cups.

BLUEBERRY DRESSING

- 1 cup blueberries (fresh or frozen)
- 1 tbsp lemon juice

Blend all ingredients until smooth.
Yields 1 cup.

Pâtés, Dips, and Spreads

These recipes are very versatile and make excellent staples. Pâtés, dips, and spreads are easy to take to work for your lunch. They're also delicious in sushi rolls, collard or romaine wraps, in sauces, and served with dehydrated crackers and veggie sticks.

Please note that nut and seed dishes will slow down the cleansing process. They are to be eaten as side dishes. Eat in small amounts, especially if you wish to lose weight.

COCONUT BUTTER

A rich spread, delicious on dehydrated crackers.

- ½ cup pure coconut oil
- 2 tbsp raw agave

Mix ingredients with a butter knife. Store in glass jar in dark, cool place.

Yields ½ cup

AVOCADO MAYO

- 1 tomato, chopped
- juice of ½ lemon
- 1 avocado, peeled, seeded, and chopped
- 1 handful basil leaves
- 2 dates, pitted and chopped

Process all ingredients together in food processor. Enjoy wrapped in romaine leaves topped with sprouts!

Yields 1 cup.

RAW KETCHUP

- 1 cup fresh tomatoes
- ½ cup sun-dried tomatoes, soaked 2–4 hours in water

Blend until smooth and store in glass jar. Keeps 1 week in the fridge.

Yields 1½ cups.

DULSE TAPENADE

A quick and nutritious spread for crackers.

- ½ cup dulse flakes
- 1 tbsp olive oil
- 2 tbsp lemon juice

Mix all ingredients by hand.

Yields ½ cup.

RAW SALSA

- 8 tomatoes, chopped
- 4 stalks celery, chopped
- ½ onion, chopped
- 1 clove garlic, minced
- ½ cup minced cilantro
- 1 jalapeno pepper, seeded and minced (optional)
- juice of 2 limes

Mix all ingredients in bowl and marinate for 1 hour.

Makes 4 servings.

CREAMY SPINACH DIP

Serve with baby carrots, cauliflower, broccoli, and red peppers.

- ½ red onion, chopped
- 1 cup spinach
- 3 cloves garlic, crushed
- ½ cup raw tahini
- 4 tbsp lemon juice
- ½ tbsp Himalayan salt
- ¼ cup fresh dill
- ¼ tsp black pepper
- dash of cayenne

Blend onion in food processor, adding spinach a little at a time. Blend with rest of ingredients until creamy.

Makes 4 servings.

AVOCADO DIP

Serve with baby carrots, red peppers, and cucumbers.

- 1 avocado, peeled and seeded
- 1 tomato, chopped
- small handful cilantro
- juice of ½ lemon
- ¼ tsp dulse

Blend all ingredients in food processor.

Makes 2 servings.

PESTO

Toss with raw zucchini noodles made in the spiral slicer or, if necessary, cooked whole grain pasta. This pesto is also excellent as a stuffing for raw mushroom caps.

• 2 cloves garlic, crushed
• 1 bunch fresh basil leaves
• ¼ cup hemp seeds
• 1 tsp Himalayan sea salt
• ¼ cup olive oil
• 2 tbsp water (optional)

Blend all ingredients well in food processor. If pesto is too thick, thin with water.

Makes 2–4 servings.

NO BEAN HUMMUS

• 3 zucchini, chopped
• 2 cloves garlic, crushed
• ½ cup raw tahini
• ¼ cup olive oil
• ¼ cup lemon juice
• ½ tsp Himalayan salt
• dash of cayenne

In food processor, blend until smooth. Garnish with fresh parsley.

Makes 4 servings.

SUNNY PÂTÉ

This is an excellent starter recipe. The lemon and garlic will help preserve it for 6 days in the fridge. For different flavors, add onion, red pepper, celery, dulse, miso, cilantro, curry, etc. Experiment and enjoy!

• 2 cups sunflower seeds, soaked overnight
• ½ cup lemon juice
• 2 cloves garlic, chopped
• 1 tbsp Nama Shoyu, unpasteurized miso, or tamari sauce
• dulse or Celtic or Himalayan salt, to taste
• 2–4 tbsp water (for consistency)

Process sunflower seeds with rest of the ingredients until smooth. If too thick, add water. Store in a covered container in the fridge. Add raw chopped vegetables, or use as a dip, salad dressing, or spread for Salad Wrap (page 152).

Makes 6 servings.

ITALIAN PÂTÉ

- 1 cup soaked sunflower seeds
- 10 sun-dried tomatoes
- 2 tbsp olive oil (optional)
- 1 clove garlic, chopped
- small bunch fresh basil

Process all ingredients in food processor. Season to taste with dulse or Himalayan salt.

Makes 4 servings.

SUNFLOWER HERB PÂTÉ

- 2 cups sunflower seeds, soaked overnight
- 1 clove garlic, chopped
- ¼ cup fresh parsley
- 2 tbsp raw tahini
- ¼ cup lemon juice
- 2 tbsp olive oil
- 1 tsp dried basil
- dash cayenne
- Himalayan salt (or dulse) to taste

Blend all ingredients in food processor. Season to taste with dulse or Himalayan salt.

Makes 8 servings.

Entrées

"IT'S Λ WRAP!"

- 4 large romaine lettuce or collard leaves
- 1 avocado, peeled, seeded, and diced
- 1 cucumber, chopped
- 1 red pepper, seeded and chopped
- 4 tbsp fresh cilantro
- 4 handfuls sunflower greens
- juice of 1 lime

Top romaine or collard leaves with other ingredients and sprinkle each with lime juice. Roll each leaf or eat as a "boat."

Makes 2 servings.

BLT

Recipe by David Klein, PhD, author of Self Healing Colitis & Crohn's *(Living Nutrition, 2005). No bacon, no bread—the B is for Brazil!*

- 1 oz sun-dried tomatoes, soaked in water
- ½ cup of Brazil nuts, soaked and ground (cashews can also be used)
- 6 large lettuce leaves
- ¼ cup pine nuts, soaked
- 1 large tomato
- 3 thin slices sweet onion (optional)

Drain sun-dried tomatoes, then blend with Brazil nuts. Add water as needed to make a workable mixture. Form the tomato mixture into 3 patties and place one on each of 3 lettuce leaves.

Drain, rinse, and blend pine nuts. Add water as needed to create a creamy consistency. Spoon the pine nut mixture over the patties. The pine nuts act like a mayonnaise.

Top each patty with a tomato slice, a slice of onion, and a leaf of lettuce.

Makes 3 servings.

ALMOND BUTTER AND BANANA SANDWICH

- 4 ripe bananas, peeled
- 4 romaine lettuce leaves
- 4 tsp raw almond butter

Spread 1 tsp of almond butter on each lettuce leaf. Place 1 banana on top and wrap leaf around it. If preferred, bananas can be mashed and spread on leaves.

Makes 4 servings.

SALAD WRAP

- 1 cup Sunflower Herb Pâté (page 151)
- 1 tomato, sliced
- 2 romaine lettuce leaves
- 2 handfuls sprouts of your choice

Spread pâté on leaves. Top with 1 tomato slice and handful of sprouts.

Makes 2 servings.

CHILI

- 1 clove garlic, chopped
- ¼ cup onion, diced
- ½ cup sun-dried tomatoes, soaked 2 hours in water
- 3 cups tomatoes, diced small
- ¾ cup zucchini, chopped
- 2 cups red pepper, seeded and diced small
- 1 cup carrots, chopped finely
- 2 tbsp chili powder
- ½ tsp cumin
- 1 tsp Italian seasoning

Process garlic, onion, sun-dried tomatoes, 2 cups tomatoes, and zucchini in food processor, blending well. Place remaining tomatoes and carrots in large bowl, then mix in blended tomato sauce. Add spices and mix well.

Makes 4 servings.

BETTER-THAN-BEANS

This recipe makes a great-tasting spread with a consistency similar to refried beans.

- 2 cups sunflower seeds, soaked
- ½ med. onion, chopped
- 2 tomatoes, chopped
- ½ cup celery, chopped
- 4 tbsp flax, hemp, or olive oil
- 1 tbsp onion powder
- 2 tsp chili powder
- 1 tsp cumin powder
- 1 tsp Himalayan salts
- 1 tbsp unpasteurized dark miso
- 1 tsp apple cider vinegar
- ¼–½ cup purified water

Blend sunflower seeds, tomatoes, and celery in a food processor. Add remaining ingredients and process again.

Makes 4–6 servings.

TOMATO MARINARA SAUCE

Use to top zucchini "noodles" made from a spiral slicer.

- 1 cup sun-dried tomatoes, soaked until soft (about 30 minutes), with the soaking water
- 2 cups chopped fresh tomatoes
- 3 tbsp olive oil
- 1 tbsp lemon juice
- 2 tbsp minced fresh oregano
- 2 tbsp Nama Shoyu
- 1 tsp fresh rosemary
- ½ tsp fresh thyme
- 1 to 2 cloves garlic
- 4–6 med. zucchini (spiralized into noodles—approximately one zucchini per serving)

Blend all ingredients—except zucchini—until smooth. Pour over "noodles" and serve.

Makes 4 servings.

STIR-NO-FRY

- ½ cup grated carrots
- ½ cup grated zucchini
- ½ cup grated daikon radish
- 1 head bok choy, chopped
- ½ cup seeded, diced red pepper
- ½ cup finely chopped red cabbage
- 1 head broccoli, finely chopped
- ½ cup roughly chopped snow pea pods
- ¼ cup green onions, chopped
- 1 tbsp raw sesame seeds (black or white)

Dressing:
- ⅓ cup lemon juice
- ⅓ cup Nama Shoyu
- 8 cloves garlic, crushed
- 1½-inch piece ginger, 1½-inch thick, peeled
- 1¼ cup olive oil.

Mix all ingredients in a large bowl. Toss with dressing and let marinate 4 hours.

Makes 4 servings.

NORI ROLLS

Nori rolls are a great fast food. Include leftover pâté for a more substantial roll. These are best made just before serving as the nori sheets quickly become soggy.

- 2 nori sheets (black sheets are usually raw)
- 1 avocado, peeled, seeded, and mashed
- 1 carrot, grated
- 1 red pepper, chopped fine
- 1 English cucumber, sliced thinly lengthwise
- sunflower, alfalfa, radish and/or clover sprouts

Spread mashed avocado on nori roll. Top with veggies and sprouts and roll the nori away from you, sealing the edge with a little water. Serve immediately.

Makes 1–2 servings.

MASHED "POTATOES"

- ⅔ cup macadamia nuts, soaked 30 minutes
- 2 cups chopped cauliflower
- ¼ cup lemon juice
- 2 tbsp olive oil
- 1 clove garlic or ¼ tsp garlic powder
- 1 tsp rosemary or Italian seasoning
- Himalayan salt and pepper, to taste

Grind nuts in food processor. Add cauliflower and remaining ingredients and blend well. Makes 2–4 servings.

Desserts

The following desserts are fairly light and won't slow down the detox process too much. Enjoy!

PRUNE DELIGHT

- 5 dates, pitted (soaked for 2 hours)
- 5 large prunes, pitted (soaked for 2 hours)
- ½ cup water
- 1 or 2 ripe bananas, peeled and sliced

Blend soaked dates and prunes with water to a smooth consistency. Serve over sliced bananas.

Makes 2 servings.

FLAX-ATIVE

A filling cereal that acts like a gentle laxative—good to eat in the morning. Chia seeds may also be used in this recipe.

- ¼ cup golden flax seeds, soaked overnight
- 1 banana, peeled
- 2 prunes, soaked (optional)
- 1 cup warm water
- ½ tsp cinnamon
- stevia to taste (optional)

Blend all ingredients.

Makes 2–4 servings.

BANANA "ICE CREAM"

My family's favorite dessert. Better than any soft ice cream!

- 4 cups frozen bananas, peeled and chopped in pieces
- 1–2 tbsp water or almond milk (optional)

Place frozen bananas in blender, food processor, or Champion juicer with the blank blade. If using blender, add just enough water or almond milk to turn bananas through the blades. Serve immediately.

Makes 2–4 servings, depending on how hungry you are!

FROZEN VANILLA BLISS

- 1 cup water
- 1 tbsp raw tahini
- 2 frozen bananas, peeled
- 1 tsp vanilla extract

In blender, combine all ingredients and blend well. Serve immediately.

Makes 2 servings.

APPLE SAUCE

- 4 gala apples, peeled, cored, and chopped
- ½ cup purified water (or Rejuvelac)
- 6 dates, pitted
- ⅛ tsp cinnamon
- pinch of nutmeg

Blend all ingredients until smooth.

Makes 2–4 servings.

CAROB CREAM

- 1 avocado, peeled and seeded
- ½ cup raw carob powder
- 2 tbsp coconut oil
- 2 tbsp raw agave

In food processor, process all ingredients until creamy.
Makes 2 servings.

CAROB PUDDING

- 1 avocado, peeled and seeded
- 1 banana, peeled
- ½ cup carob powder
- 2–3 dates, pitted and soaked

Blend all ingredients in food processor until creamy.
Makes 2 servings.

CASHEW CREAM

Delicious and rich—to be eaten in moderation.

- 1 cup cashew nuts, soaked
- 1 cup purified water (or Rejuvelac)
- 4 gala apples, peeled, cored, and chopped
- 6 dates, pitted (soaked 2–4 hours)

Blend all ingredients together until smooth.
Makes 4 servings.

DECADENT CHOCOLATE SAUCE

A tasty topping for "banana ice cream" or as a fondue!

- 1 tbsp raw carob powder
- 1 tsp raw tahini
- ½ tsp coconut oil
- 2 tsp raw agave
- dash of cinnamon

Blend all ingredients until smooth.
Makes 2 servings.

BANANA PUDDING

- 6 ripe bananas, peeled
- ½ cup fresh apple juice (or water)
- 1½ cups raisins
- ¼ tsp nutmeg
- 2 tbsp raw agave

Blend all ingredients until smooth. Refrigerate until chilled.

Makes 2–4 servings.

RAW APPLE PIE

Crust:
- 3 cups almonds, chopped
- 1 cup dates, pitted

In food processor, process until dough sticks together. Press into 8-inch pie dish.

Filling:
- 6 apples, chopped finely
- 2 tbsp lemon juice
- dash cinnamon
- 1 tbsp psyllium powder
- ½ cup fresh blueberries, raspberries, or other berries for garnish (optional)

Process 2 apples in food processor with lemon juice and psyllium powder. Place in bowl with remaining apples. Mix by hand and add to pie shell. Decorate pie slices with fresh berries if you wish.

Makes 8 servings.

FUSS-FREE CARROT CAKE

A delightful carrot cake with a guilt-free "cream cheese" icing!

- 6 medium carrots, chopped
- 2 large apples, peeled and chopped
- 1 cup dried apricots, soaked 1 hour
- 1 cup raisins, soaked 1 hour
- 1 cup dried coconut
- 1 tsp cinnamon
- ½ tsp dried ginger
- ½ tsp ground nutmeg
- ¼ tsp cardamom
- ½ tsp orange zest

In a food processor, process carrots and apples. Transfer to bowl. Next, process apricots and raisins, adding to the carrot mixture. Mix in the remaining ingredients by hand. Press into spring form pan and refrigerate while preparing the icing.

CASHEW CHEESE ICING

- 1 cup raw cashews, soaked 4 hours
- ½ cup purified water
- 2 tbsp raw agave
- juice of 1 lemon
- 2 tbsp shredded coconut

Blend cashews with water, agave, and lemon juice until creamy, adding more water if necessary. Spread icing on cake and top with shredded coconut.

Makes 8 servings.

Recommended Reading and Resources

BOOKS

Airola, Paavo. *Are You Confused?* Health Plus Publishing, 1971.

Anderson, Rich. *Cleanse & Purify Thyself—The Clean Me Out Program*. Rich Anderson, 1992.

Anderson, Rich. *The Rave Diet & Lifestyle. ravediet.com*, 2004.

Boutenko, Victoria. *Green for Life*. Raw Family Publishing, 2005.

Boutenko, Victoria. *12 Steps to Raw—How to End Your Dependency on Cooked Food*. North Atlantic Books, 2007.

Brazier, Brendan. *The Thrive Diet: The Whole Food Way to Lose Weight, Reduce Stress, and Stay Healthy*. Da Capo Press, 2007.

Campbell, Colin T. and Thomas M. Campbell II. *The China Study: The Most Comprehensive Study of Nutrition Ever Conducted*. Benbella Books, 2006.

Clement, Brian. *Hippocrates LifeForce*. Healthy Living Publications, 2007.

Cousens, Gabriel. *Conscious Eating*. North Atlantic Books, 2000.

Diamond, Harvey. *Fit for Life, Not Fat for Life*. Health Communications Inc., 2003.

Dorit. *Celebrating Our Raw Nature*. Book Publishing Company, 2007.

Hay, Louise. *Heal Your Body*. Hay House, 1984.

Meyerowitz, Steve. *Sproutman's Kitchen Garden Cookbook*. Sproutman Publications, 1999.

Meyerowitz, Steve. *Sprouts the Miracle Food: The Complete Guide to Sprouting*. Sproutman Publications, 1998.

Monarch, Matt. *Raw Success*. Monarch Publishing, 2007.

Nison, Paul. *Raw Food Formula for Health*. Healthy Living Publications, 2008.

Rogers, Sherry A. *Detoxify or Die*. Prestige, 2002.

Stokes, Angela. *Raw Emotions*. E-book available from: *store.rawreform.com*

Vasey, Christopher. *The Acid-Alkaline Diet for Optimal Health*. Healing Arts Press, 2004.

Wigmore, Ann. *The Blending Book: Maximizing Nature's Ingredients*. Avery Publishing, 1997.

Wigmore, Ann. *The Hippocrates Diet and Health Program*. Avery Publishing, 1983.

Wigmore, Ann. *Recipes for Health and Longer Life*. Avery Publishing, 1982.

Wigmore, Ann. *The Sprouting Book—How to Grow and Use Sprouts to Maximize Your Health and Vitality*. Avery, 1986.

RECOMMENDED FILMS

Eating (*ravediet.com*, 2008).
Healing Cancer from the Inside Out (*ravediet.com*, 2008).
Vegan Fitness Built Naturally (M. Johnson Production, 2005).
You Can Heal Your Life (Hay House, 2008).

HELPFUL WEBSITES

annwigmore.org

fromsadtoraw.com

hippocratesinst.org

livingnutrition.com

nutritiondata.com

paulnison.com

ravediet.com

rawfamily.com

rawfoods.com

rawreform.com

rawspirit.org

serenityspaces.org

simplyraw.ca

sunfood.com

treeoflife.nu

Nutrient values of select greens

Eat your greens! Dark, leafy greens contain an abundance of vitamins, minerals, and antioxidants. They are rich in fiber and folic acid and are one of the richest nondairy sources of calcium. The high vitamin C and magnesium content enhances the absorption of calcium. Eating foods rich in chlorophyll (in green vegetables) also helps provide the body with vitamin K and oxygen-carrying red blood cells.

Make sure to vary your leaf choices. Below are some of the more common greens we like to add to our smoothies and salads.

Arugula (Amounts per 1 leaf, 2 g)

Calories	0.5 (2.1 kJ)	Vitamin C	0.3 mg
Protein	0.1 g	Vitamin K	2.2 mcg
Total Carbohydrate	0.1 g	Folate	1.9 mcg
Total Fat	0.0 g	Calcium	3.2 mg
Omega-3 fatty acids	3.4 mg	Magnesium	0.9 mg
Omega-6 fatty acids	2.6 mg	Phosphorus	1.0 mg
Vitamin A	47.5 IU	Potassium	7.4 mg
Beta Carotene	28.5 mcg	Sodium	0.5 mg

Source: *NutritionData.com*

Avocados (Amounts per 1 cup, 150 g)

Calories	240 (1005 kJ)	Niacin	2.6 mg
Protein	3.0 g	Vitamin B6	0.4 mg
Total Carbohydrate	12.8 g	Folate	122 mcg
Dietary Fiber	10.1 g	Calcium	18.0 mg
Total Fat	22.0 g	Iron	0.8 mg
Omega-3 fatty acids	165 mg	Magnesium	43.5 mg
Omega-6 fatty acids	2534 mg	Phosphorus	78.0 mg
Vitamin A	219 IU	Potassium	727 mg
Beta Carotene	93.0 mcg	Sodium	10.5 mg
Vitamin C	15.0 mg	Zinc	1.0 mg
Vitamin E	3.1 mg	Copper	0.3 mg
Vitamin K	31.5 mcg	Manganese	0.2 mg
Thiamin	0.1 mg	Selenium	0.6 mcg
Riboflavin	0.2 mg	Fluoride	10.5 mcg

Source: *NutritionData.com*

Bok choy (Amounts per 1 cup, 70 g)

Calories	9.1 (38.1 kJ)	Niacin	0.3 mg
Protein	1.0 g	Vitamin B6	0.1 mg
Total Carbohydrate	1.5 g	Folate	46.2 mcg
Dietary Fiber	0.7 g	Calcium	73.5 mg
Total Fat	0.1 g	Iron	0.6 mg
Omega-3 fatty acids	35.7 mg	Magnesium	13.3 mg
Omega-6 fatty acids	27.3 mg	Phosphorus	25.9 mg
Vitamin A	3128 IU	Potassium	176 mg
Beta Carotene	1877 mcg	Sodium	45.5 mg
Vitamin C	31.5 mg	Zinc	0.1 mg
Vitamin E	0.1 mg	Manganese	0.1 mg
Vitamin K	25.1 mcg	Selenium	0.3 mcg

Source: *NutritionData.com*

Celery (Amounts per 110 g)

Calories	17.6 (73.7 kJ)	Vitamin B6	0.1 mg
Protein	0.8 g	Folate	39.6 mcg
Total Carbohydrate	3.3 g	Choline	6.7 mg
Dietary Fiber	1.8 g	Calcium	44.0 mg
Total Fat	0.2 g	Iron	0.2 mg
Omega-6 fatty acids	86.9 mg	Magnesium	12.1 mg
Vitamin A	494 IU	Phosphorus	26.4 mg
Beta Carotene	297 mcg	Potassium	286 mg
Vitamin C	3.4 mg	Sodium	88.0 mg
Vitamin E	0.3 mg	Zinc	0.1 mg
Vitamin K	32.2 mcg	Manganese	0.1 mg
Riboflavin	0.1 mg	Selenium	0.4 mcg
Niacin	0.4 mg	Fluoride	4.4 mcg

Source: *NutritionData.com*

Cilantro (Amounts per ¼ cup 4 g)

Calories	0.9 (3.8 kJ)	Vitamin E	0.1 mg
Protein	0.1 g	Vitamin K	12.4 mcg
Total Carbohydrate	0.1 g	Folate	2.5 mcg
Dietary Fiber	0.1 g	Calcium	2.7 mg
Total Fat	0.0 g	Iron	0.1 mg
Omega-6 fatty acids	1.6 mg	Magnesium	1.0 mg
Vitamin A	270 IU	Phosphorus	1.9 mg
Alpha Carotene	1.4 mcg	Potassium	20.8 mg
Beta Carotene	157 mcg	Sodium	1.8 mg
Vitamin C	1.1 mg		

Source: *NutritionData.com*

Collard greens (Amounts per 1 cup, chopped 36 g)

Calories	10.8 (45.2 kJ)	Vitamin K	184 mcg
Protein	0.9 g	Niacin	0.3 mg
Total Carbohydrate	2.0 g	Vitamin B6	0.1 mg
Dietary Fiber	1.3 g	Folate	59.8 mcg
Total Fat	0.2 g	Calcium	52.2 mg
Omega-3 fatty acids	38.9 mg	Iron	0.1 mg
Omega-6 fatty acids	29.5 mg	Magnesium	3.2 mg
Vitamin A	2400 IU	Phosphorus	3.6 mg
Alpha Carotene	85.7 mcg	Potassium	60.8 mg
Beta Carotene	1383 mcg	Sodium	7.2 mg
Vitamin C	12.7 mg	Manganese	0.1 mg
Vitamin E	0.8 mg	Selenium	0.5 mcg

Source: *NutritionData.com*

Cucumber (Amounts per ½ cup slices 52 g)

Calories	7.8 (32.7 kJ)	Niacin	0.1 mg
Protein	0.3 g	Folate	3.6 mcg
Total Carbohydrate	1.9 g	Choline	3.1 mg
Dietary Fiber	0.3 g	Calcium	8.3 mg
Total Fat	0.1 g	Iron	0.1 mg
Omega-3 fatty acids	2.6 mg	Magnesium	6.8 mg
Omega-6 fatty acids	14.6 mg	Phosphorus	12.5 mg
Vitamin A	54.6 IU	Potassium	76.4 mg
Alpha Carotene	5.7 mcg	Sodium	1.0 mg
Beta Carotene	23.4 mcg	Zinc	0.1 mg
Vitamin C	1.5 mg	Selenium	0.2 mcg
Vitamin K	8.5 mcg	Fluoride	0.7 mcg

Source: *NutritionData.com*

Dandelion greens (Amounts per 1 cup, chopped, 55 g)

Calories	24.7 (103 kJ)	Niacin	0.4 mg
Protein	1.5 g	Vitamin B6	0.1 mg
Total Carbohydrate	5.1 g	Folate	14.9 mcg
Dietary Fiber	1.9 g	Calcium	103 mg
Total Fat	0.4 g	Iron	1.7 mg
Omega-3 fatty acids	24.2 mg	Magnesium	19.8 mg
Omega-6 fatty acids	144 mg	Phosphorus	36.3 mg
Vitamin A	2712 IU	Potassium	218 mg
Beta Carotene	1628 mcg	Sodium	41.8 mg
Vitamin C	19.3 mg	Zinc	0.2 mg
Vitamin E	2.6 mg	Copper	0.1 mg
Vitamin K	151 mcg	Manganese	0.2 mg
Thiamin	0.1 mg	Selenium	0.3 mcg
Riboflavin	0.1 mg		

Source: *NutritionData.com*

E$_3$Live (per 1 g)

Calories	260cal/100g	Calcium	14.0 mg
Protein	60 %	Chloride	0.47 mg
Carbohydrate	12%	Chromium	0.53 mcg
Omega-3 fatty acids	29.50 mg	Cobalt	2.0 mcg
Omega-6 fatty acids	6.00 mg	Copper	4.30 mcg
Ascorbic Acid C	6.70 mcg	Fluoride	38.0 mcg
Biotin	0.33 mcg	Iodine	0.53 mcg
Choline	2.30 mcg	Iron	350.7 mcg
Cobalimin B12	8.00 mcg	Magnesium	2.20 mg
Folic Acid	1.00 mcg	Manganese	32.0 mcg
Inositol	0.35 mcg	Molybdenum	3.30 mcg
Niacin B3	0.13 mcg	Nickel	5.30 mcg
B5	6.80 mcg	Phosphorus	5.20 mcg
Beta carotene	1890 IU	Potassium	12.0 mcg
Pyridoxine B6	11.1 mcg	Selenium	0.67 mcg
Riboflavin B2	49 mcg	Silicon	186.5 mcg
Thiamine B1	4.80 mcg	Sodium	2.70 mg
Vitamin E	0.13 IU	Tin	0.47 mcg
Vitamin K	40.0 mcg	Titanium	46.60 mcg
Boron	0.15 mg	Zinc	18.7 mcg

Source: *NutritionData.com*

Kale (Amounts per 1 cup, chopped, 67 g)

Calories	33.5 (140 kJ)	Vitamin B6	0.2 mg
Protein	2.2 g	Folate	19.4 mcg
Total Carbohydrate	6.7 g	Calcium	90.5 mg
Total Fat	0.5 g	Iron	1.1 mg
Omega-3 fatty acids	121 mg	Magnesium	22.8 mg
Omega-6 fatty acids	92.4 mg	Phosphorus	37.5 mg
Vitamin A	10302 IU	Potassium	299 mg
Beta Carotene	6182 mcg	Sodium	28.8 mg
Vitamin C	80.4 mg	Zinc	0.3 mg
Vitamin K	547 mcg	Copper	0.2 mg
Thiamin	0.1 mg	Manganese	0.5 mg
Riboflavin	0.1 mg	Selenium	0.6 mcg
Niacin	0.7 mg		

Source: *NutritionData.com*

Lambsquarter (Amounts per 1 oz, 28 g)

Calories	12.0 (50.2 kJ)	Folate	8.4 mcg
Protein	1.2 g	Calcium	86.5 mg
Total Carbohydrate	2.0 g	Iron	0.3 mg
Dietary Fiber	1.1 g	Magnesium	9.5 mg
Total Fat	0.2 g	Phosphorus	20.2 mg
Omega-3 fatty acids	10.1 mg	Potassium	127 mg
Omega-6 fatty acids	87.6 mg	Sodium	12.0 mg
Vitamin A	3248 IU	Zinc	0.1 mg
Vitamin C	22.4 mg	Copper	0.1 mg
Riboflavin	0.1 mg	Manganese	0.2 mg
Niacin	0.3 mg	Selenium	0.3 mcg
Vitamin B6	0.1 mg		

Source: *NutritionData.com*

Mustard greens (Amounts per 1 cup, 56 g)

Calories	14.6 (61.1 kJ)	Niacin	0.4 mg
Protein	1.5 g	Vitamin B6	0.1 mg
Total Carbohydrate	2.7 g	Folate	105 mcg
Dietary Fiber	1.8 g	Calcium	57.7 mg
Total Fat	0.1 g	Iron	0.8 mg
Omega-3 fatty acids	10.1 mg	Magnesium	17.9 mg
Omega-6 fatty acids	11.2 mg	Phosphorus	24.1 mg
Vitamin A	5881 IU	Potassium	198 mg
Beta Carotene	3528 mcg	Sodium	14.0 mg
Vitamin C	39.2 mg	Zinc	0.1 mg
Vitamin E	1.1 mg	Copper	0.1 mg
Vitamin K	278 mcg	Manganese	0.3 mg
Riboflavin	0.1 mg	Selenium	0.5 mcg

Source: *NutritionData.com*

Parsley (Amounts per 1 cup, 60 g)

Calories	21.6 (90.4 kJ)	Niacin	0.8 mg
Protein	1.8 g	Vitamin B6	0.1 mg
Total Carbohydrate	3.8 g	Folate	91.2 mcg
Dietary Fiber	2.0 g	Calcium	82.8 mg
Total Fat	0.5 g	Iron	3.7 mg
Omega-3 fatty acids	4.8 mg	Magnesium	30.0 mg
Omega-6 fatty acids	69.0 mg	Phosphorus	34.8 mg
Vitamin A	5055 IU	Potassium	332 mg
Beta Carotene	3032 mcg	Sodium	33.6 mg
Vitamin C	79.8 mg	Zinc	0.6 mg
Vitamin E	0.4 mg	Copper	0.1 mg
Vitamin K	984 mcg	Manganese	0.1 mg
Thiamin	0.1 mg	Selenium	0.1 mcg
Riboflavin	0.1 mg		

Source: *NutritionData.com*

Romaine lettuce (Amounts per 1 inner leaf, 6 g)

Calories	1.0 (4.2 kJ)	Vitamin K	6.2 mcg
Protein	0.1 g	Folate	8.2 mcg
Total Carbohydrate	0.2 g	Choline	0.6 mg
Dietary Fiber	0.1 g	Calcium	2.0 mg
Total Fat	0.0 g	Iron	0.1 mg
Omega-3 fatty acids	6.8 mg	Magnesium	0.8 mg
Omega-6 fatty acids	2.8 mg	Phosphorus	1.8 mg
Vitamin A	348 IU	Potassium	14.8 mg
Beta Carotene	209 mcg	Sodium	0.5 mg
Vitamin C	1.4 mg		

Source: *NutritionData.com*

Spinach (Amounts per 1 cup, 30 g)

Calories	6.9 (28.9 kJ)	Niacin	0.2 mg
Protein	0.9 g	Vitamin B6	0.1 mg
Total Carbohydrate	1.1 g	Folate	58.2 mcg
Dietary Fiber	0.7 g	Calcium	29.7 mg
Total Fat	0.1 g	Iron	0.8 mg
Omega-3 fatty acids	41.4 mg	Magnesium	23.7 mg
Omega-6 fatty acids	7.8 mg	Phosphorus	14.7 mg
Vitamin A	2813 IU	Potassium	167 mg
Beta Carotene	1688 mcg	Sodium	23.7 mg
Vitamin C	8.4 mg	Zinc	0.2 mg
Vitamin E	0.6 mg	Manganese	0.3 mg
Vitamin K	145 mcg	Selenium	0.3 mcg
Riboflavin	0.1 mg		

Source: *NutritionData.com*

Swiss chard (Amounts per 1 cup, 36 g)

Calories	6.8 (28.5 kJ)	Niacin	0.1 mg
Protein	0.6 g	Folate	5.0 mcg
Total Carbohydrate	1.3 g	Calcium	18.4 mg
Dietary Fiber	0.6 g	Iron	0.6 mg
Total Fat	0.1 g	Magnesium	29.2 mg
Omega-3 fatty acids	2.5 mg	Phosphorus	16.6 mg
Omega-6 fatty acids	22.7 mg	Potassium	136 mg
Vitamin A	2202 IU	Sodium	76.7 mg
Alpha Carotene	16.2 mcg	Zinc	0.1 mg
Beta Carotene	1313 mcg	Copper	0.1 mg
Vitamin C	10.8 mg	Manganese	0.1 mg
Vitamin E	0.7 mg	Selenium	0.3 mcg
Vitamin K	299 mcg		

Source: *NutritionData.com*

About SimplyRaw

I believe that the living foods lifestyle can change people's lives for the better, and I have seen many people transform their health by adopting a raw and living foods diet. During 2004, I made the decision to launch my own business, SimplyRaw, as a way to reach out to the public and help educate people. SimplyRaw is my passion, my belief, and an expression of my life. I am excited to be helping people experience well-being and increased health, and to observe the transformations that the living foods lifestyle can bring to peoples' lives.

SimplyRaw is primarily serviced-based. We offer live food preparation workshops, focusing on quick and easy recipes that maximize nutritional value. SimplyRaw also offers raw food chef certification classes and natural weight loss programs based on my eighteen years of experience with the living foods lifestyle.

My detox program has evolved and developed since 2006. The program provides either monthly group participation or personalized individual detox coaching worldwide. This manual is based on the constructive feedback from thousands of detox group participants who contributed to its constant evolution and refinement.

Community involvement is very important to me and my family. We reach out and engage the community as often as possible. Since 2004 we have organized monthly raw vegan potlucks, with over fifty people in regular attendance, and about 120 people at our largest potluck (excluding our raw wedding potluck which attracted approximately 160 people). The SimplyRaw Festival is now the largest free raw vegan festival in North America (and possibly the world). Starting in 2006 as an idea to promote the raw lifestyle through a raw pie contest, it was a half-day event. The 2008 event brought together over fifty exhibitors, dozens of renowned speakers from across North America, and thousands of delighted participants over the course of the weekend. Giving to the community is important for my husband and me, and SimplyRaw regularly participates in a variety of free community events, whether health shows, environment fairs, music festivals, food fairs, or street parties.

Recipes in **bold**.

A

acid-alkaline diet, 105–106
Acid-Alkaline Diet by Christopher Vasey, 106
acidic foods *(table)*, 106
affirmations, positive and SRLFD, 64
alfalfa tea, 113
alkaline foods *(table)*, 106
Almond Butter and Banana Sandwich, 152
animal protein, 41. *See also* plant protein
Ann Wigmore's Energy Soup. *See also*
    Energy Soup, 135
Apple Sauce, 156
Apple-Kale Green Smoothie, 121
apples in Energy Soup, 36
Avocado Dip, 149
Avocado Mayo, 148
avocados in Energy Soup, 36

B

Banana "Ice Cream," 156
Banana Pudding, 129, 158
Banana Shake, 119
Banana-Avocado Pudding, 127
Banana-Mango-Spinach Pudding, 130
Banana-Spinach Green Smoothie, 48
beauty products. *See* personal care products
    and skin care products
bee pollen, 112
Berry Smoothie, 120
Better-than-Beans, 153
Blended Salad, 139
blending in Week 4 (Days 3,4,5), 87
blending and juicing of raw foods, 39–40
BLT, 152
Blue Bliss Pudding, 129
Blueberry Dressing, 147
Blueberry Milkshake, 126
Bosc Pear-Raspberry-Kale Green
    Smoothie, 48
Breakfasts (recipes), 131–133
breakfasts, raw in SRLFDP, 68
breathing, deep, 95
buckwheat greens/sprouts in Energy Soup,
    36
Buckwheat Porridge, 131
burdock root tea, 113

C

Cabbage Rejuvelac. *See also* **Rejuvelac**
    ingredients and preparation, 38
Cabbage Slaw, 144
caffeine, 70–71. *See also* coffee
calcium, 110
Carob Cream, 157
Carob Pudding, 157
Carob Shake, 120
Carob Super-Shake, 126
Carob-Date Shake, 125
Carrot-Apple Shake, 119
Cashew Cheese Icing, 159
Cashew Cream, 157
cat's claw tea, 113
cayenne tea, 113
chamomile tea, 113
chemicals, 19–20. *See also* toxins
    in cleaning products, 60
    in personal care products, 62
chewing and digestion, 26, 68
chia seeds, 112
children and detox program, 57
Chili, 153
China Study, The by T. Colin Campbell, 42
chlorella, 111
Citrus Drink, 118
cleaning products, 60
cleansing. *See* detoxification
cleansing reactions, 30–31
    during Week 3, 84
Coconut Butter, 148
coffee. *See also* caffeine
    withdrawal from, 70–71
colon cleansing, 96. *See also* colonic irrigation
colonic irrigation, 96–97
    in Week 3, 83
    in Week 4, 86
colonics. *See* colonic irrigation
cooked foods
    harmful effects of, 24
Cool Cucumber Soup, 137
cosmetics. *See* skin care products and personal
    care products
cravings, food, 56–57, 82
Cream of Tomato Soup, 135
Cream of Zucchini Soup, 133
Creamy Cauliflower Soup, 137
Creamy Celery Soup, 134
Creamy Italian Dressing, 145
Creamy Kale Soup, 136
Creamy Pear Pudding, 128